SACRED THREADS EXHIBITION 2013

Quilts Exploring Joy, Inspiration, Peace, Grief, Healing and Spirituality

Lauren Kingsland, Editor

Acknowledgements

Cover art: A Tree of Life by Lin Schiffner, Nevada City, CA, USA

Sacred Threads 2013 Organizing Committee members:
Lisa Ellis, Chairman, Annabel Ebersole, Sandi Goldman, Barbara Hollinger, Susanne Jones, Bunnie Jordan, Lauren Kingsland, Audrey Lipps, Vivian Milholen, Carole Nichols, Shana Spiegel, Anne Winchell.

All artwork used by permission of the artists. Photography and text provided by the artists.

Special thanks to Ruthie Lindal Swain for her editorial assistance.

www.sacredthreadsquilts.com

In cooperation with CQS Press, Gaithersburg, MD 20878

ISBN:0978704428
ISBN-13:978-0978704421

CONTENTS

About the show

Sacred Threads 2013 was a national juried exhibition of 231 quilts from 195 artists exploring themes of joy, inspiration, peace/brotherhood, grief, healing and spirituality,. The show was held July 10 - July 28, 2013, at Floris United Methodist Church, 13600 Frying Pan Road, Herndon, VA, 20171.

The quilts in **Sacred Threads 2013** present an artistic look at the deeper side of life. The themes of joy, inspiration, peace and brotherhood, grief, healing and spirituality are addressed through visual stories by these artists. There are pieces made as responses to the shootings at Sandy Hook, about coping with Alzheimer's in a loved one, and of coming through an illness back to health. There are celebrations of the beauty of the Earth and of our common humanity around the world. There are colorful, gorgeous expressions of spirituality and religious devotion from a variety of faith traditions.

In its 10th year, this biennial exhibition offers a respectful, dignified venue for the artwork of quilters of all faiths who use their work as a connection to the sacred and/or as an expression of their spiritual journey. These powerful stories-in-fabric from quilt artists throughout the USA and Canada offer an inspiring source of encouragement, healing, strength and connection.

For more information go to www.sacredthreadsquilts.com.

JOY

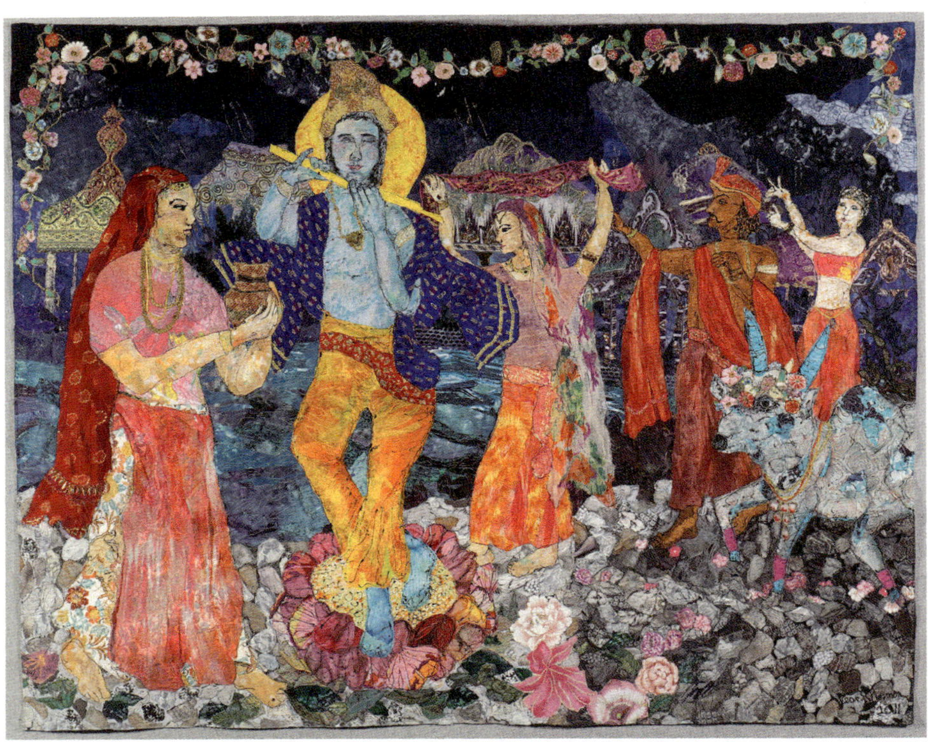

Jean Herman Denver, CO, USA
Krishna Brings the Rain 55” x 42”

Throughout history human kind has looked for God's blessing on our crops and has asked God to send rain. "Krishna Brings the Rain" honors this tradition by showing the joy of the dancers as they dance and play music asking their Hindu God Shiva to bring rain. Hindu culture is based on many of these joyful traditions that celebrate life and the blessings from the Gods. I hope this piece embodies the beauty and joy found in this ancient rite.

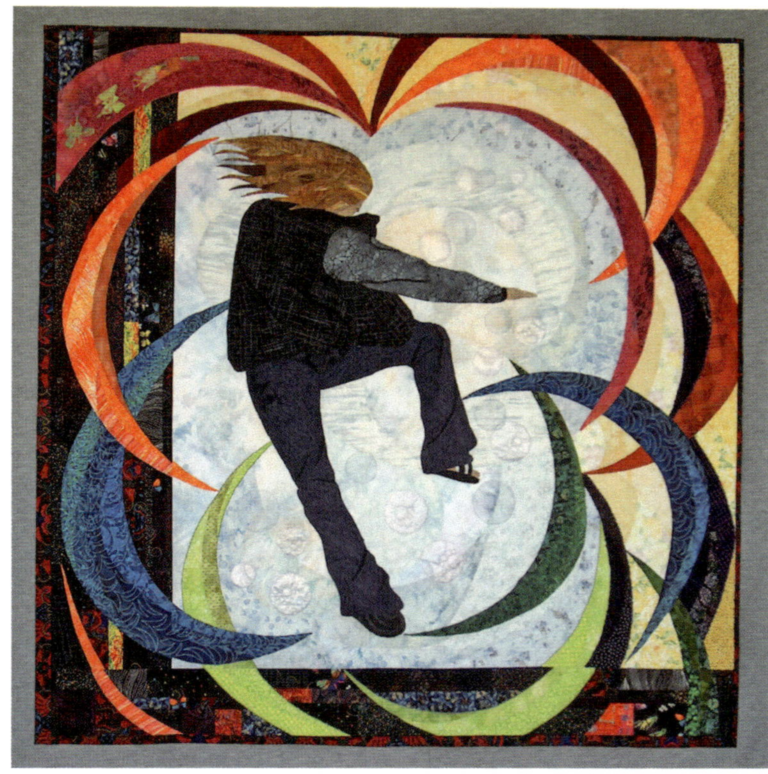

Wendy Butler Berns
Lake Mills, WI, USA

Pure Joy, Imagine That
51" x 51"

Ahhh, to frolic with jubilant mirth and delight
for no other reason than just for the pure pleasure of it.
Imagine that!!

Growing older often stifles our playful spirit.
Our wisdom makes us cautious. We wonder what others will think of our actions.
We surround ourselves with little black clouds of doubt.

Can we find that passion and exuberant feeling again?
Let's try. Just imagine...pure joy!

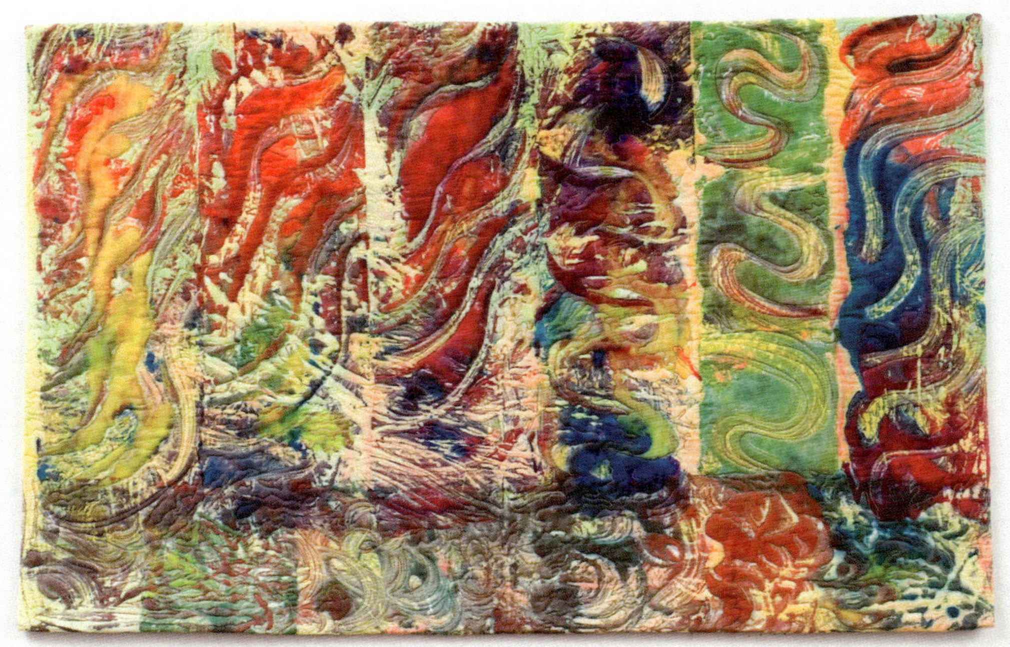

Benedicte Caneill Larchmont, NY, USA
Dance of the Spirits 33" x 21"

The Native American Cree people have called Aurora Borealis or Northern Lights the "Dance of the Spirits". Northern Lights dance through the sky to remind the living people that the spirits of their loved ones are watching over them. In the Middle Ages the auroras were believed to be a sign from God. Whatever the belief is, they do remain a fantastic sight. This piece is not meant to literally depict an aurora but rather evoke the inspiring and soul-lifting joy of this phenomenon.

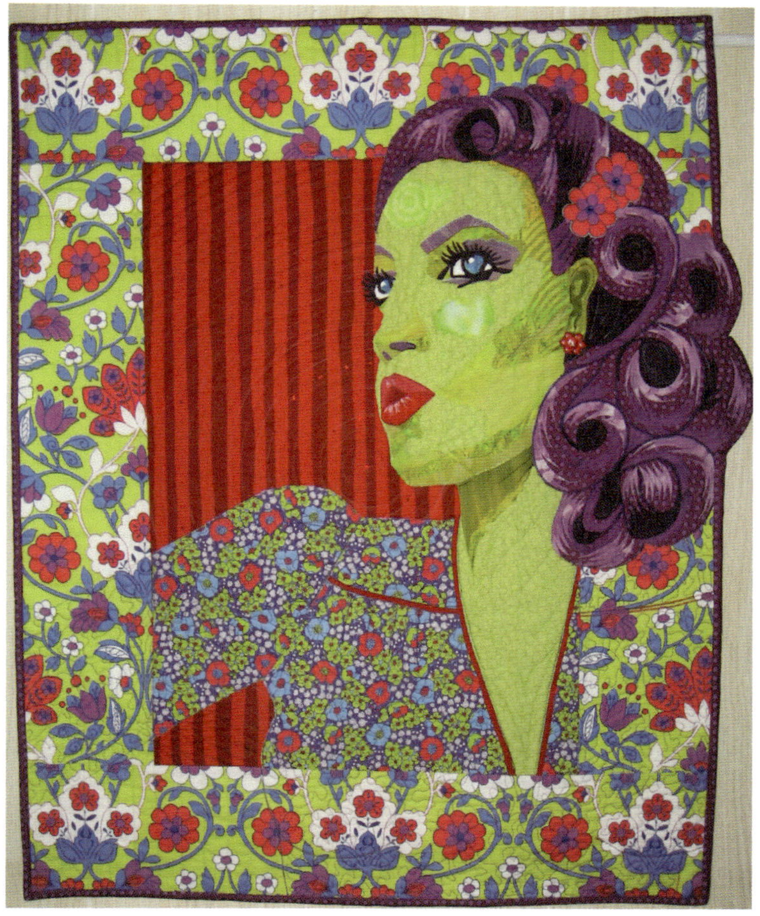

Laurie Ceesay
Menominee, MI, USA

Victory Rolls
28" x 35"

I am a fiber artist and a hairdresser and I find extreme joy in using my knowledge and enthusiasm of hair designs and vintage hairstyles to create portrait quilts with this process. I am intrigued by the hairstyles of the 1940s and began this quilt with excitement! I was able to visit a friend in Florida last winter and found the bright lime floral at the local quilt shop. When I look at the quilt I am reminded of this awesome quilt store in Winter Haven, Florida! I found great joy in using the bright colors of the large scale print to design this project. I felt like I was stepping back in time and reviewing my cosmetology textbook with pin curl technical examples. I enjoyed using my 1940s paper doll book to inspire me with the fashions of the decade.

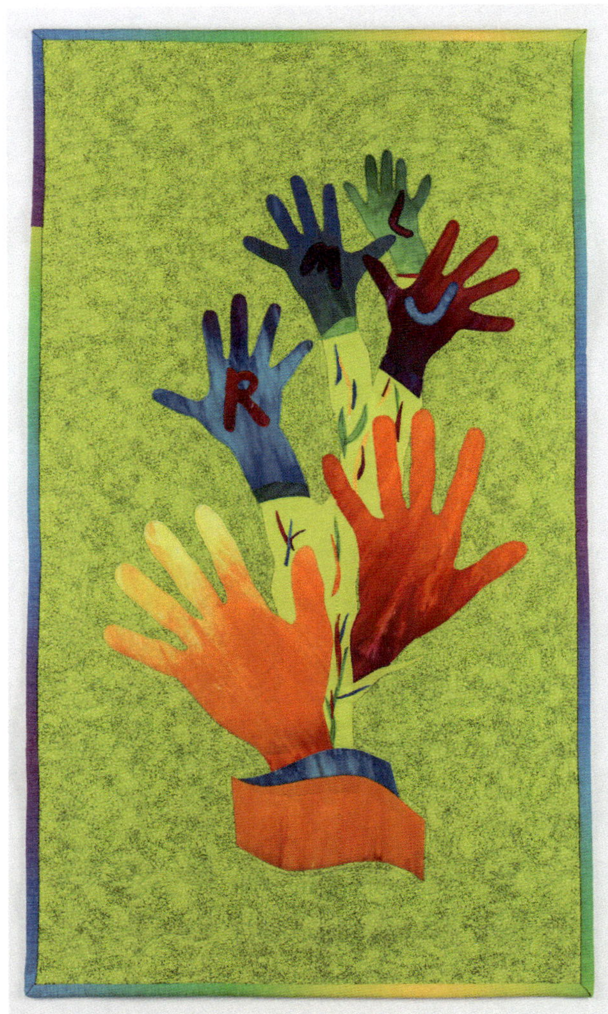

Charlotte Jackson
Fort Collins, CO, USA

Grandparent's Family Tree
18.25" x 31"

This piece was inspired by a Six Word Poem that I wrote: "Yours, Mine, Ours, Theirs, Grandparents Finally!" It celebrates the great joy in being a grandma, and my immense love for our four cherished grandchildren. Each small hand, while physically traced onto the quilt, also symbolizes the place that child holds etched into my heart. The capacity for love is limitless--every opportunity to do so enlarges and extends the path of my life's journey.

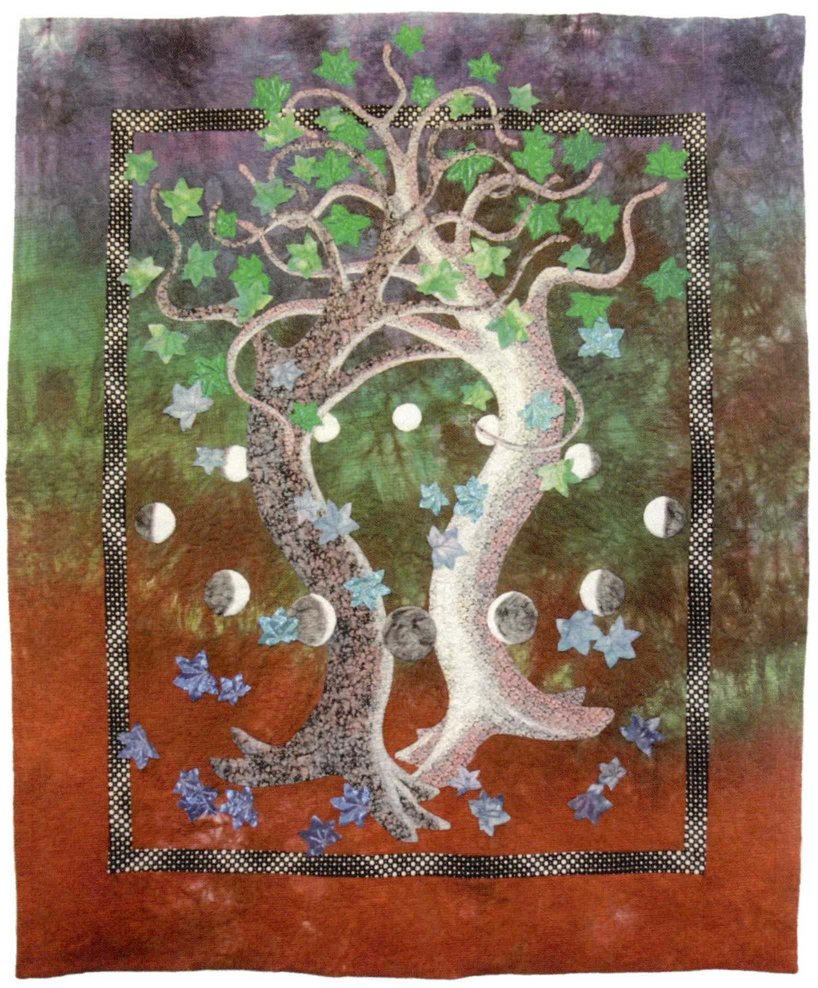

Eileen Doughty
Vienna, VA, USA

Moon Dance
42" x 51"

This was inspired by Van Morrison's song, "Moon Dance." Light from an invisible source shines on the trees. These are not tame trees.

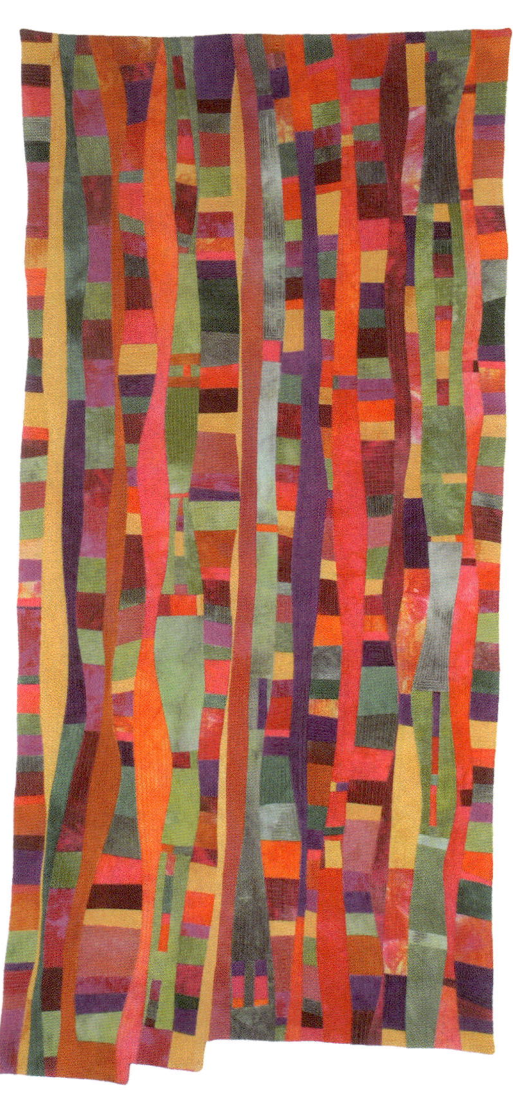

Susan Schrott
Mount Kisco, NY, USA

Andantino
21"x 45"

BRFWA...Breathe, Relax, Feel, Watch and Allow the joy to fill our lives. With a passionately beating heart reflecting an abundance of movement and colors we are blessed to take actions in service of our values and are free to do so with fluidity and mindfulness.

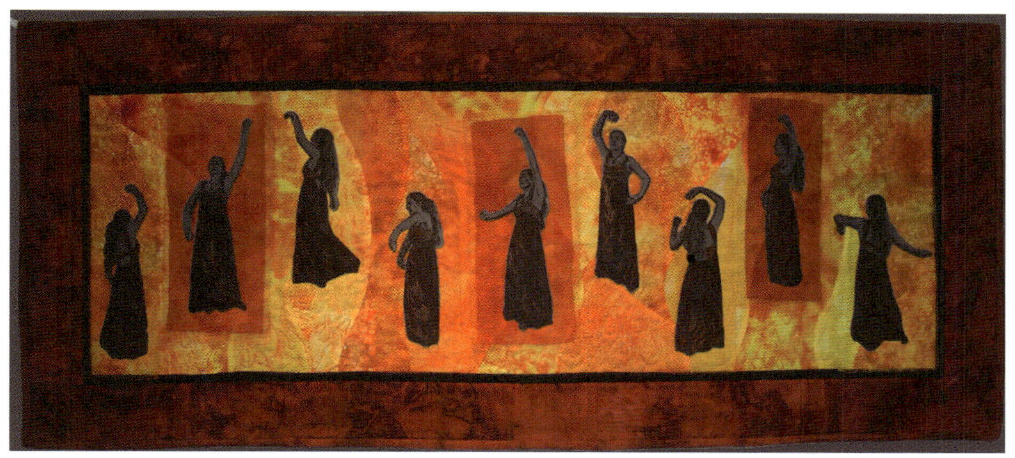

Lisa A Arthaud Warrenton, VA, USA
Girl On Fire 52" x 22 "

"Mom, Mom! Guess What!" My 13 year old daughter's class finished reading Hunger Games and all students had to create final projects based on the book. She was determined to create her own "Girl On Fire" dress, complete with flickering flames.

The sewing room was soon ablaze in glowing red, orange and yellow fabrics.
Fortitude. Passion. Tenacity. Creativity. As she twirled in her finished handiwork, her tacked on flame-shaped organza fluttered wildly about her.

"Mom, I did it!" Exuberance. Pride. Joy. Using her dress scraps, I recreated the moment and printed her sewing pattern onto the border.

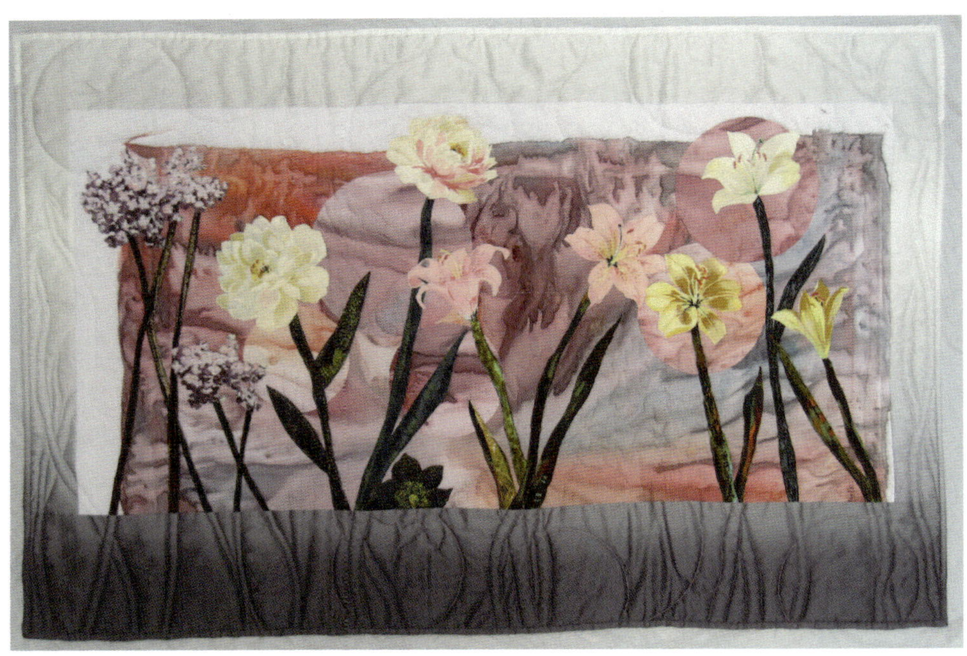

Linda T. Cooper Burke, VA, USA
Joy 48" x 31"

When I couldn't figure out how to use the much-larger pink background I had painted, I gave it to my quilting friend, Joy Bauer, who wanted to make a whole-cloth quilt. Joy died in 2011 and her son, John gave it back to me. We have so many good intentions in life and only a limited time to accomplish them. Just like the flowers in the quilt, Joy bloomed brightly and lived up to her name. I was pleased to make this quilt and when I see it I remember Joy.

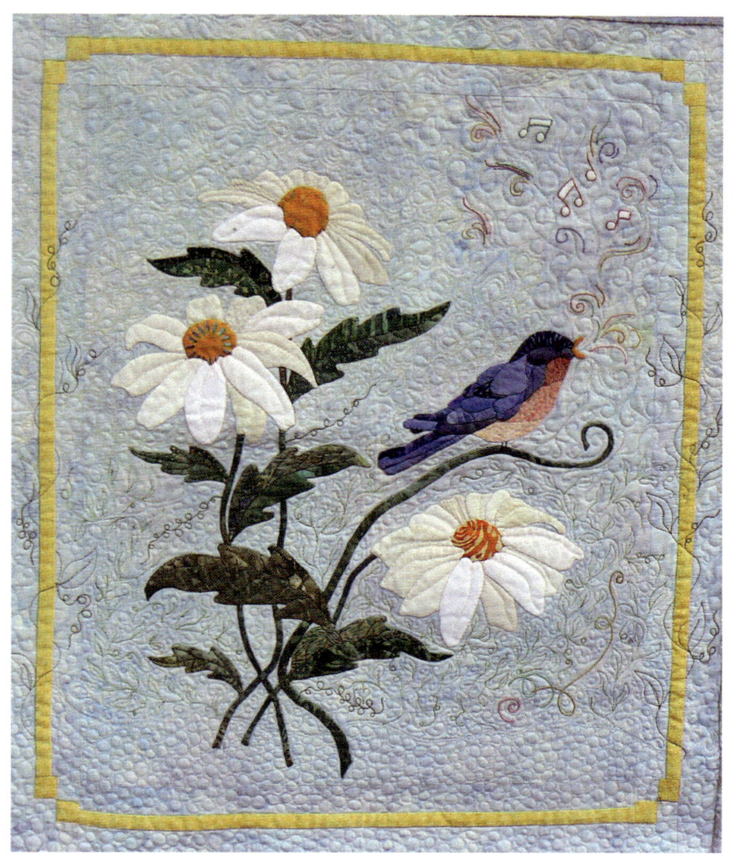

Jo Moury
Haymarket, VA, USA

Joyful Noise
24" x 29"

The inspiration for the joyous little bird singing in the early morning light came from the cover art on a Sunday Bulletin. Thinking of this happy little fellow singing praises to the Lord just makes me happy. I wish we all could sing His praises with such abandon. In the words of my favorite praise hymn: "He is exalted, the King is exalted on high. I will praise Him. He is exalted; forever exalted and I will praise His name".

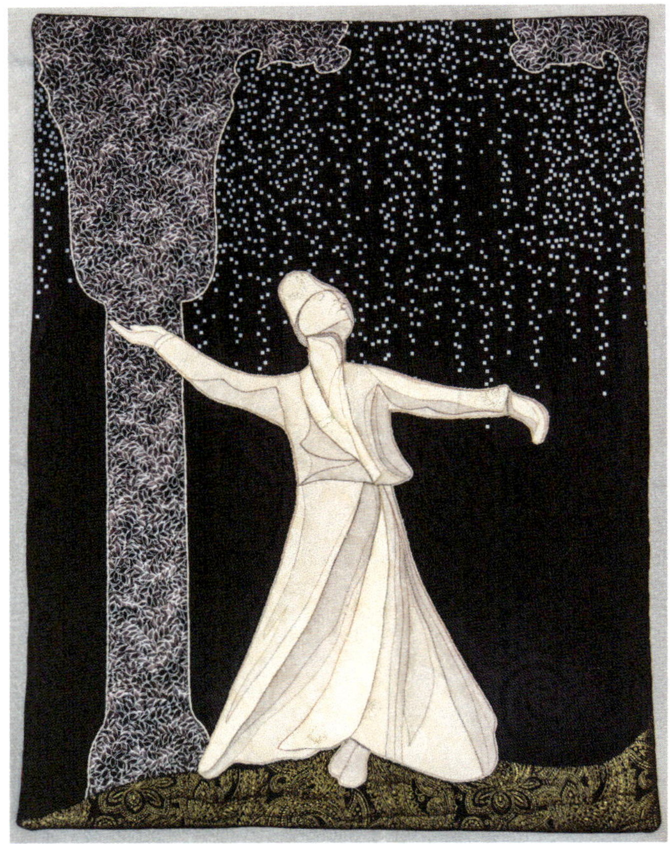

Connie L Smyer
Chandler, AZ, USA

Turn to Joy of Existence
20.5" x 27"

In the Spring of 2012, I was fortunate to observe a demonstration of practicing Dervishes "Turning" - what we in the West refer to as whirling. The Turning took place in a restored caravanserai near Konya, Turkey, the home and burial place of the famed Sufi poet, Rumi (Jelaluddin Balkhi). Rumi introduced Turning to the Mevlevi Dervish community in the 13th Century. Originally an expression of Rumi's grief over the loss of a dear friend, "Turning" is at once meditative, prayer-like and peaceful. Above all it is a joyous dance celebrating life itself.

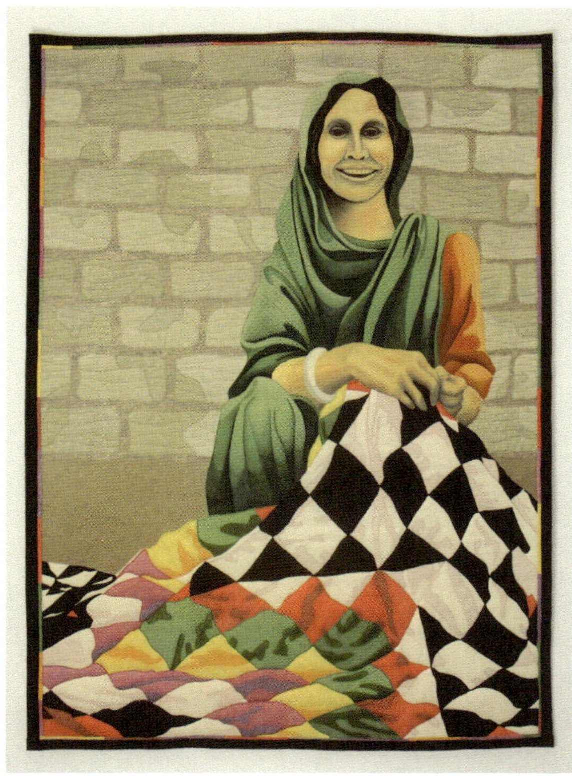

Linda Anderson
La Mesa, CA, USA

Threads of Identity
34" x 46"

I have lived in a country where many women have very limited opportunities for choices in Life that we Westerners think are necessary for experiencing Joy and fulfillment. This woman is her family's constant caretaker, and making quilts out of whatever is available brings her joy and satisfaction. Caretaking is her identity, and the joy she sews into each and every quilt and garment is her strength and legacy for the next generation.

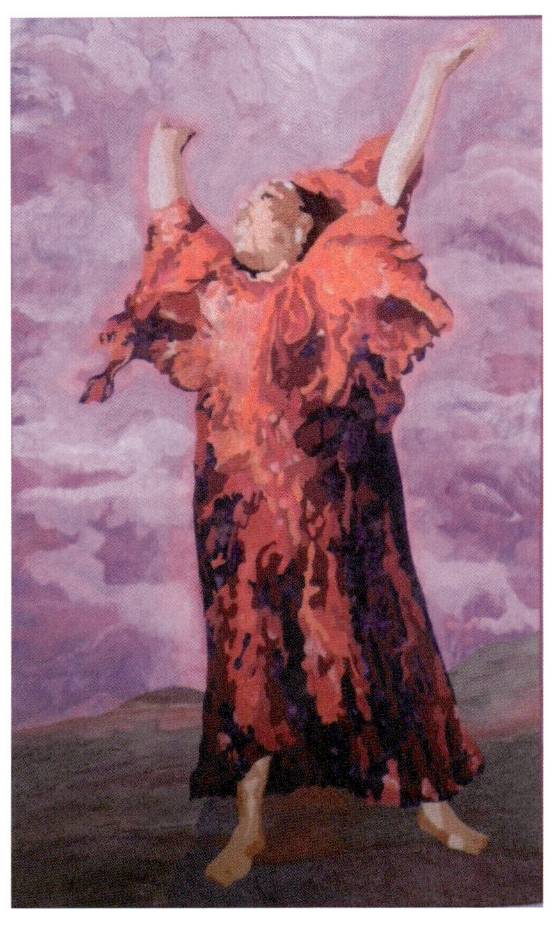

Sandy Curran
Newport News, VA, USA

HALLEUJAH
42" x 68"

A number of years ago, after a life of teaching exercise for a living, I began to slowly loose my mobility. At first the pain was bearable. Later, I had to quit teaching. Finally, I could not walk or perform the most basic tasks. After successful surgery, I have my mobility back. But more than that, I have my identity and sense of self back. This gift is more wonderful than anything except my husband and my daughter. I am so joyously grateful, I walk every day and thank God for the ecstasy of pain free movement and the physical ability to be outside in the beauty of nature. Hallelujah! There are many parts of your life you cannot appreciate till you lose them.

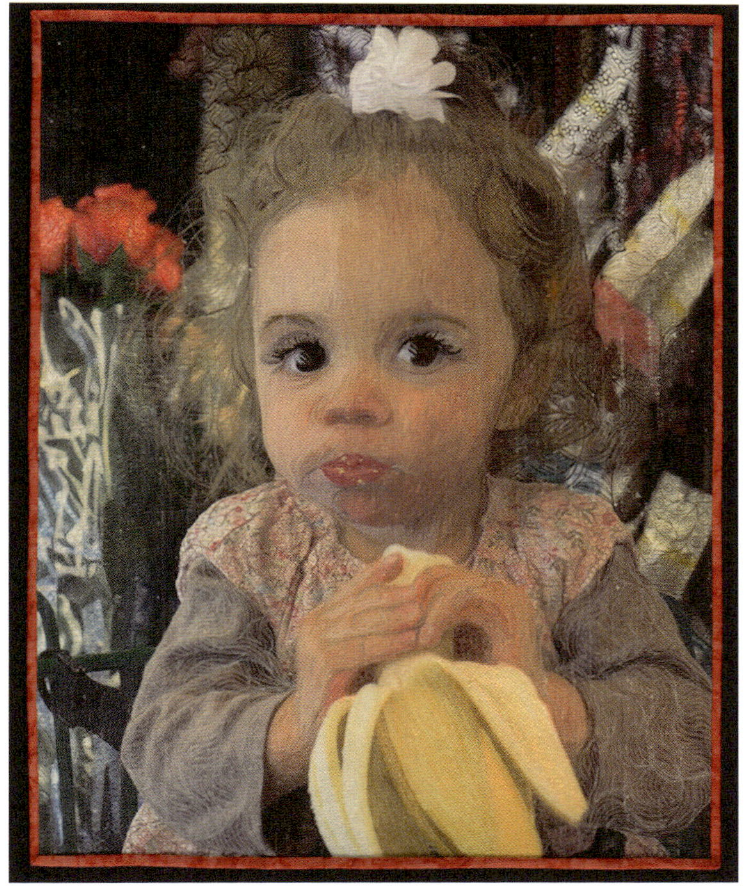

Jennifer Day
Santa Fe, NM, USA

Mmmm....Good
22" x 27"

"Mmmm...Good" is a quilt made from a photograph that I took of a three year old girl eating a banana in her shopping cart at the grocery. You know that the banana was the most important thing in her life at that moment and it tasted sooo...good! What a joy that her grandmother pulled it off the rack for her to eat!!!! The joy in the faces of children is what we look forward to every day.

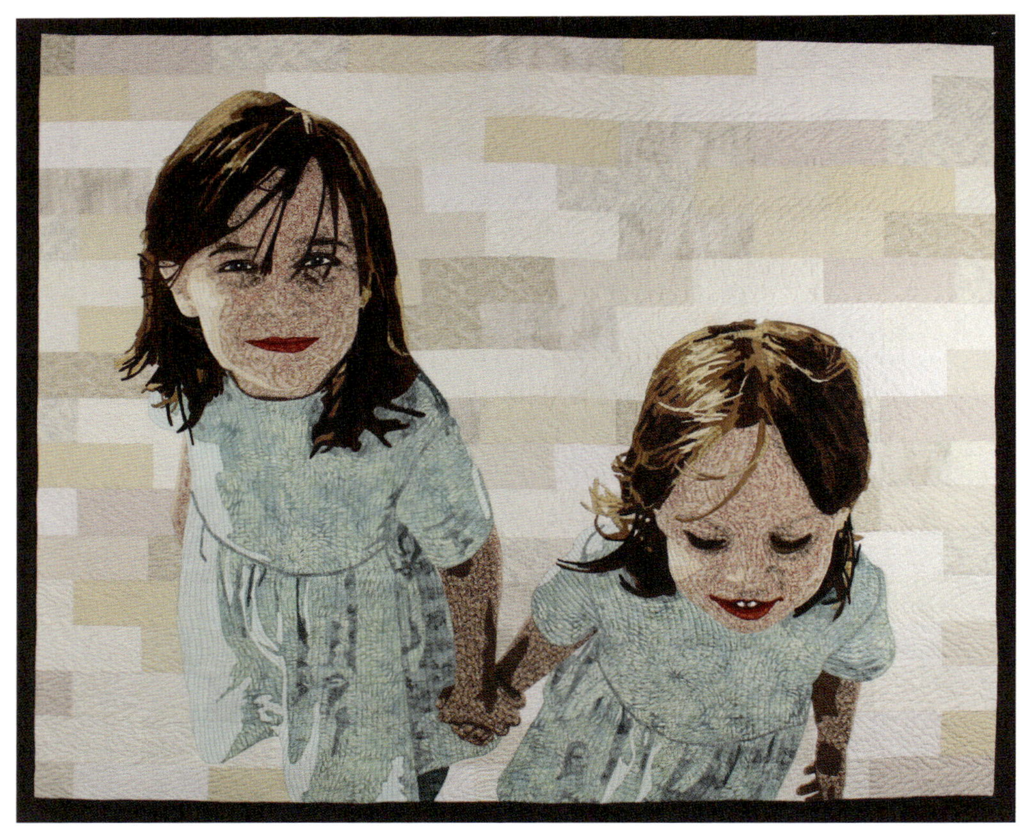

Virginia S. Greaves Roswell, GA, USA
Beach Guardians 42" x 33"

Children are the ultimate joy of our lives for those that are willing to have the eyes to see. There is nothing more moving than when they look up into our faces with trust and happiness.

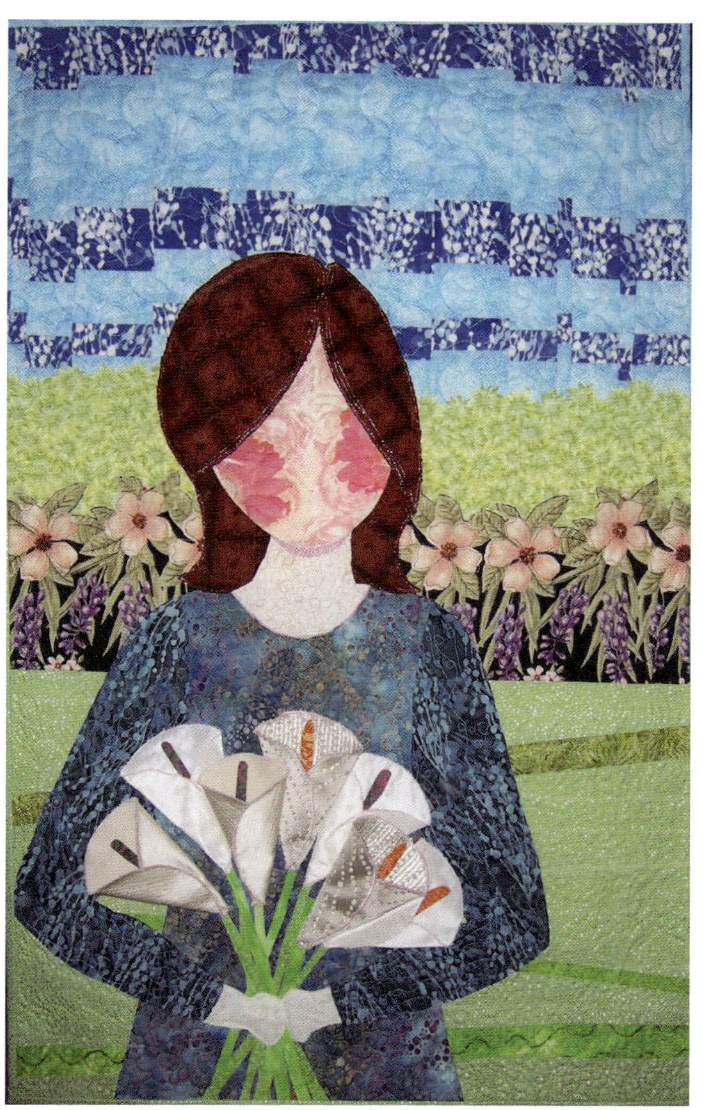

Ann E Turley
Fallbrook, CA, USA

Consider the Lilies
22.5" x 35"

Christ asks us in Luke 12:27 to "Consider how the lilies grow...not even Solomon in all his splendor is dressed like these." God beautifully clothes the grasses of the field, yet His own glory outshines everything. What joy I feel when I consider His great love for us and the grace that gloriously covers all of His children.

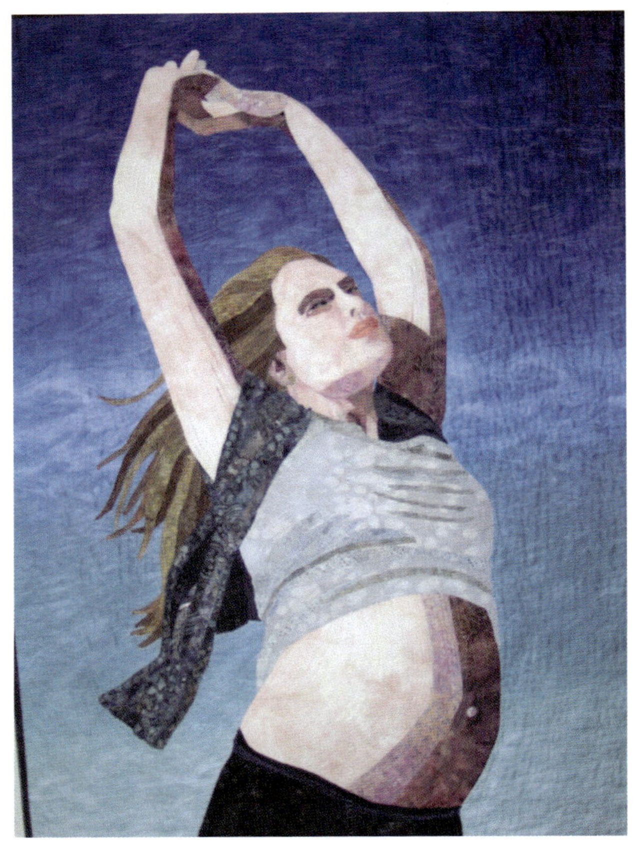

Barbara A Allen
Colorado Springs, CO, USA

33 Weeks
39” x 44”

My quilt is all about sanctity of ife. What greater joy has God given us? "For you created my inmost being; you knit me together in my mother's womb. I praise you because I am fearfully and wonderfully made; your works are wonderful, I know that full well. My frame was not hidden from you when I was made in the secret place, when I was woven together in the depths of the earth. Your eyes saw my unformed body; all the days ordained for me were written in your book before one of them came to be." Psalm 139:13-16.

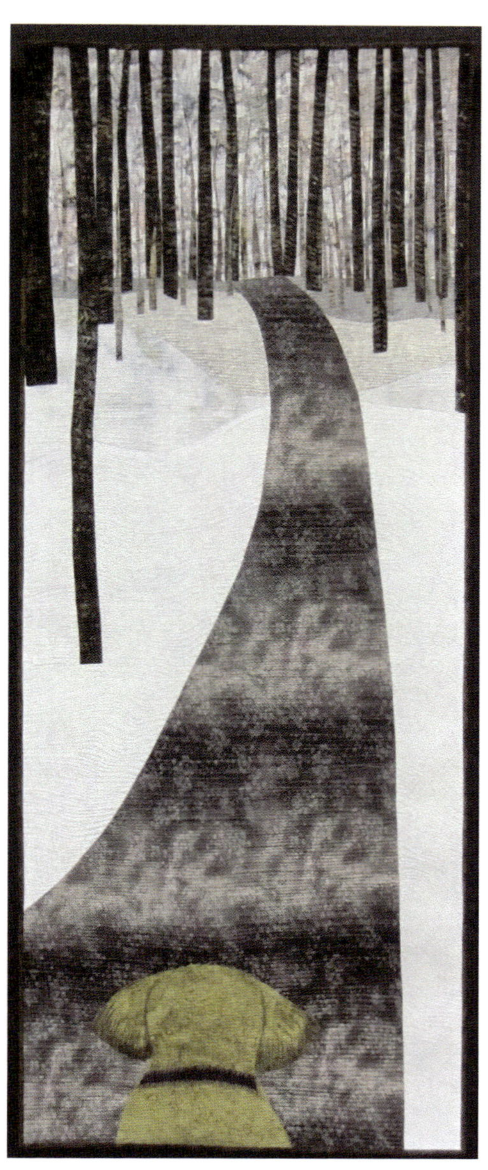

Cyndi Z Souder
Annandale, VA, USA

Let's Go!
24" x 59"

Our 11-year-old Chesapeake Bay Retriever looks forward to our afternoon walks. If I'm working in my studio when it's time for her walk, Rowan the Wonderdog comes to find me. She especially likes to take walks in the cold weather. She oozes joy, prancing in the snow with her ears flapping in the breeze. I find her joy contagious; her celebration encourages me to embrace the moment and leave my worries behind.

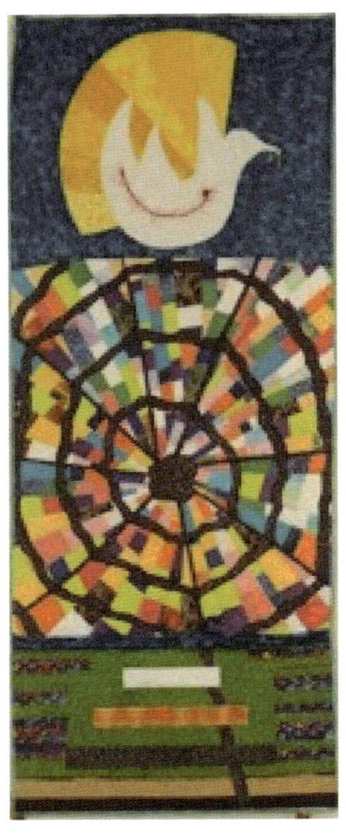

Laura Comiskey Broders
New Orleans, LA, USA

The New Rings of Life at Easter
32 x 67”

This Easter banner is in a liturgical series for the St. Ignatius Chapel at Loyola University, New Orleans, Louisiana.

The Calvary cross on which Jesus was crucified extends down into the earth from which the felled tree was taken to construct the cross, represented by the black printed fabric. The vertical plane of the cross meets the horizontal plane at the bottom "step" of death; the cross/death is destroyed when the vertical plane is severed on the second golden orange "step" representing the resurrection of Jesus; and the third white step representing the ascension of Jesus. The cross explodes into the rings of life of the tree surrounded by the brilliant colors in the center of the banner representing the new order in the world upon Jesus' resurrection.

The beauty, strength and gentleness of the Holy Spirit gifted to us at Jesus' ascension is represented in the dove whose body pulses with the blood of life as it carries the Word of God offering eternal salvation to all.

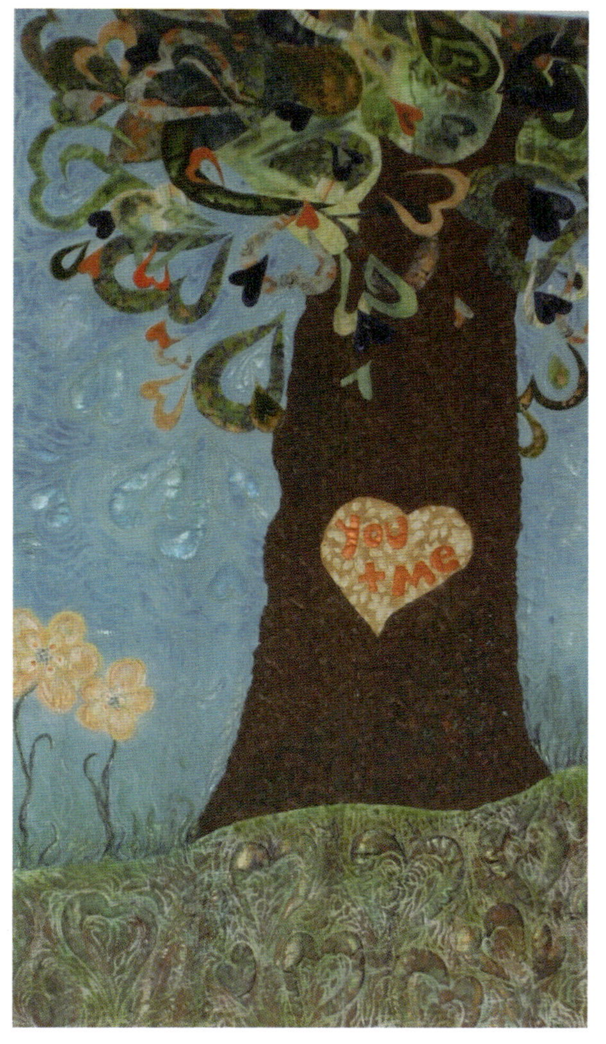

Amalia P Morusiewicz
Mitchellville, MD, USA

Rooted in the Heart
24” x 42”

Our lives are woven with connections on our spiritual journeys. Through those relationships our lives, like the texture of the bark, become more interesting. A joy shared is increased and in every story we share our hearts. My personal challenge of exploring texture was inspired by the simple beauty of tree bark.

This professes love, and connections, as we are all rooted in the heart. "You + me" invites the viewer to participate. In sharing my art, I share my joys and passion through these threads that connect us.

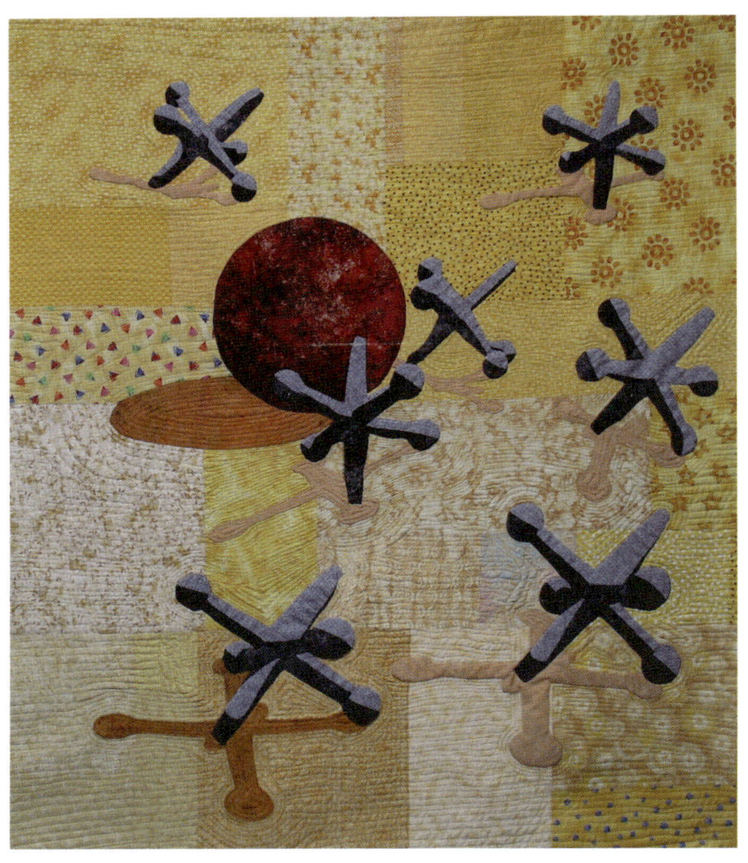

Karen S Musgrave Naperville, IL, USA

Simpler Times 46" x 52"

The goal for the summer of 1965 was to become the champion of Jacks. The competition lived next door. We had decided on Jacks because she did not want to play baseball and I did not want to play with dolls. It was not just about the game, but the adventures to find the perfect place to play. When summer ended, we decided to share the title and have a rematch the following summer. It was not to be. Diane moved so the joy of our friendship and time together became a sweet memory.

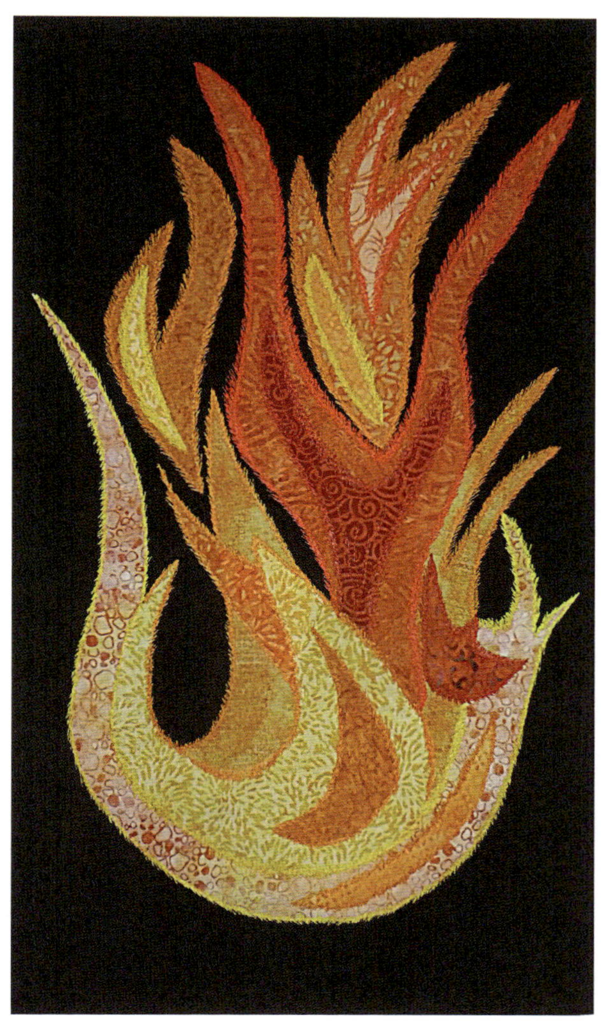

Kathy Lincoln
Burke, VA, USA

The Light of My Life
18” x 30”

My husband and I have always enjoyed a good fire in our fireplace, both the inside and outside kind. So this quilt is a reflection of one of the joys we share in our life together. We will sit in front of our fireplace and watch the flames while we talk about our day or things that we are planning. The freedom to create for me comes from being in a secure place to express myself. My art is an expression of where I am at the moment. So this quilt is dedicated to the "light of my life", my husband of almost 35 years.

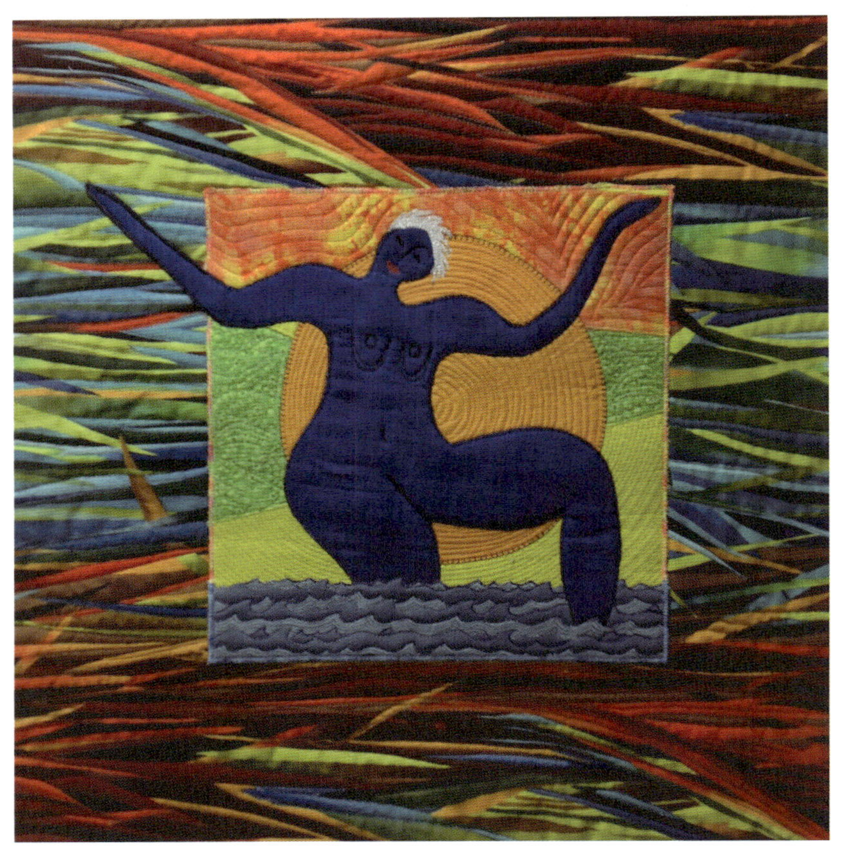

Kate Owens Conroe, TX, USA
It's Good To Be Me 21" x 21"

The journey to getting older has its benefits - it seems with each passing decade we strip away the layers that are no longer a part of who we are. Eventually we become less self-conscious and more comfortable in the skin we're in! That's when it feels good to be me!

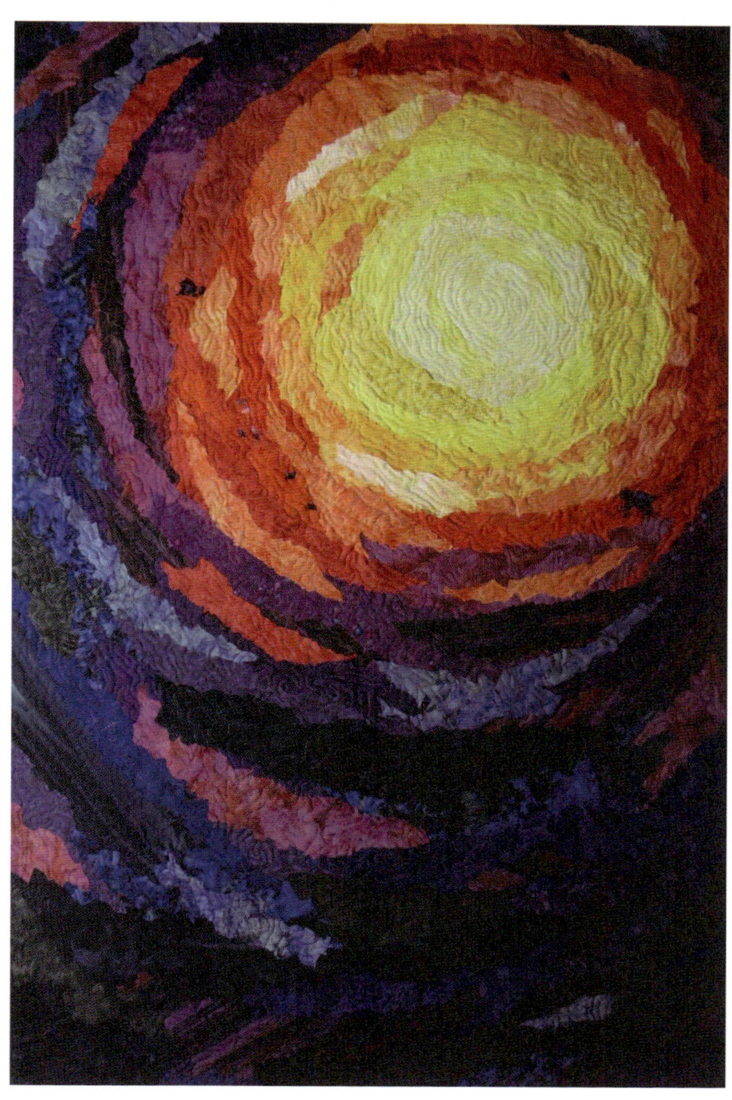

Patricia Powers
Lynchburg, VA, USA

The Heavens Sing
29” x 43”

The Easter season is one of joy as I celebrate the resurrection of Jesus. The heavens, indeed, all nature, sing His praises!

"OUR FAMILY
IS A CIRCLE
OF LOVE
AND STRENGTH
WITH EVERY
BIRTH
AND EVERY
UNION
THE CIRCLE
GROWS
EVERY JOY
SHARED
ADDS MORE
LOVE
EVERY
OBSTACLE
FACED
TOGETHER
MAKES
THE CIRCLE
STRONGER."

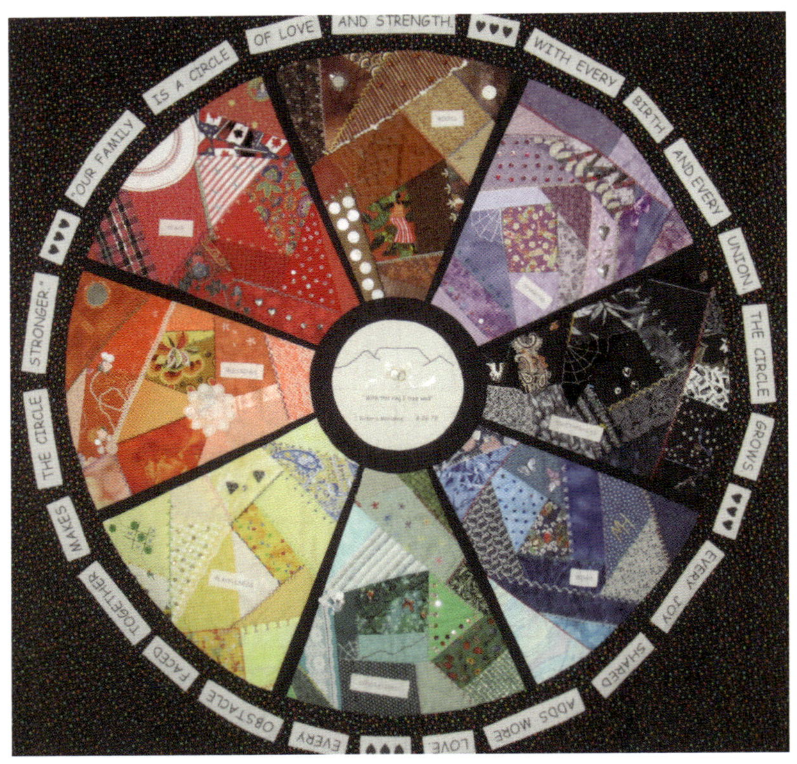

Marianne H Hendrickse Ellicott City, MD, USA

Family Circle Celebrations-Why My Rainbow Has Brown

57" x 56"

This quilt express joy and the history of our family, our origins, traditions and values. Our family is originally from South Africa, and with the different backgrounds of our children's spouses (Philipino, Salvadorian and Arab/Native American) we are truly a rainbow family. I added brown to the rainbow circle to represent our Roots where growing up under the Apartheid regime, the color of one's skin determined to a great extent where one lived, went to school and worked.

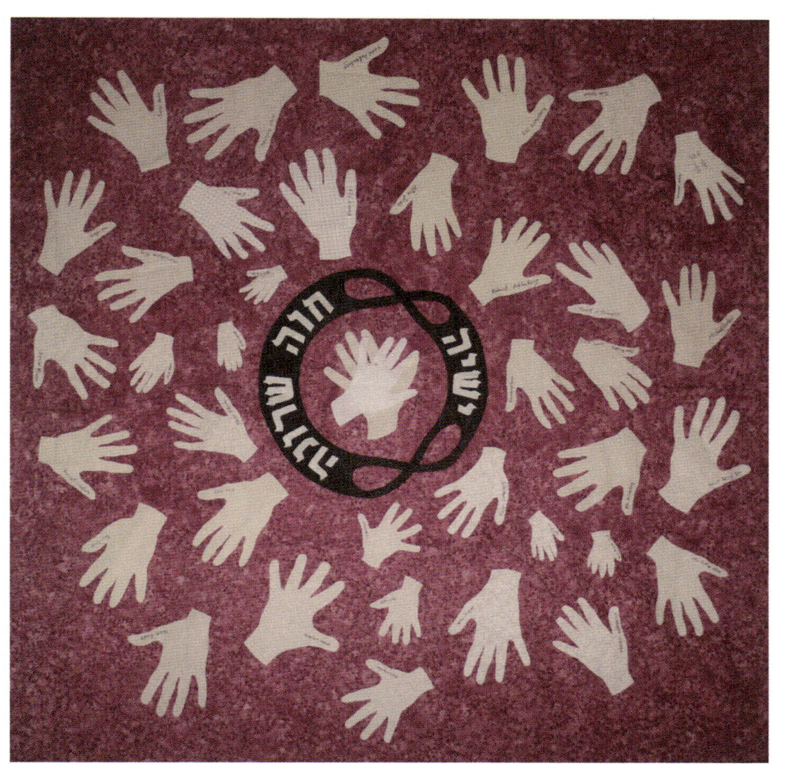

SherriJoyce King Gladwyne, PA, USA
With So Much Love 60" x 60"

This chuppah - a canopy used in Jewish weddings to symbolize the home the couple will build together - is graced with the hands and hugs of close family and friends of my niece and new nephew. Tracings of hands were sent to me from both coasts and across the ocean. Look closely... you can see that the same fabric is used for all members of each family. Sadly, both the oldest hand and the youngest passed away before the wedding... we were so glad to have their treasured love included in the chuppah. A hug stays in a quilt forever. Joy!

INSPIRATION

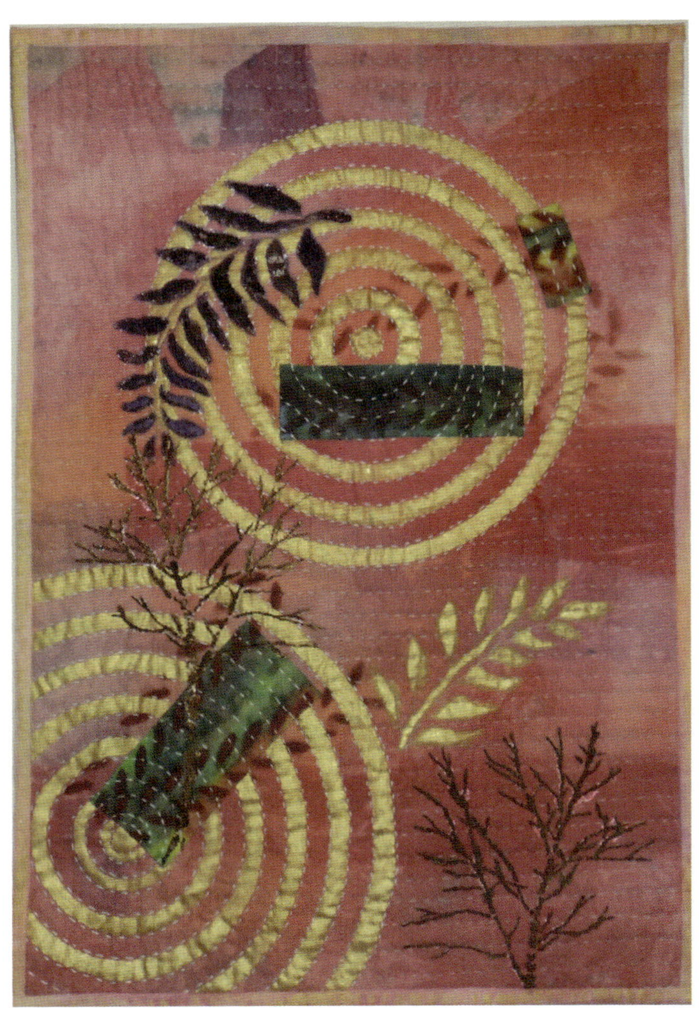

Winifred B Wallace
Silver Spring, MD, USA

Let Them Be For Lights
23" x 16"

My inspiration came from Genesis, the first book of the Bible. As part of my Creation Series this is a whole cloth interpretation of Genesis 1:15. "And let them be for lights in the firmament of the heaven to give light upon the earth: and it was so."

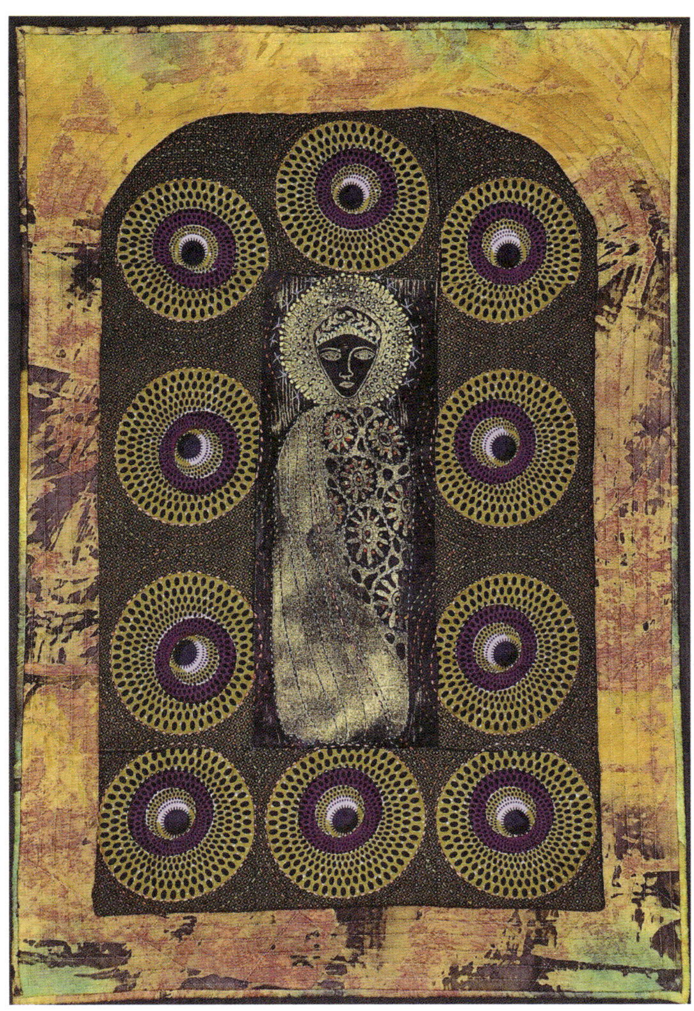

Diane Wright
Guilford, CT, USA

Sentinel
24.5" x 35"

Australian artist Dijanne Cevaal encouraged like-minded fiber artists to use her "Sentinelle" linocut in their own work. It is her hope that the figure will inspire others and stand vigil around the world, in places high and low.

Dijanne Cevaal created the central figure as a linocut.

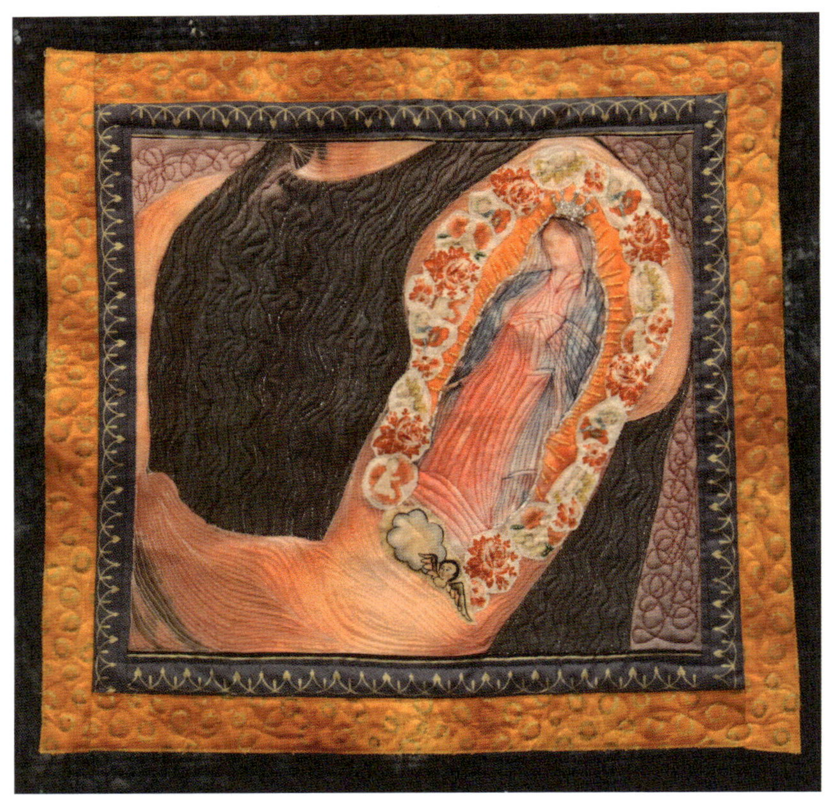

Kathy S Zieben Houston, TX, USA

Armed With Grace 24" x 23"

Our Lady of Guadalupe is an avatar of the Virgin Mary who allegedly first appeared before the peasant Juan Diego in 1531. The Virgin imprinted an image of herself surrounded by roses on his tilma, a thin blanket-type-covering made of cactus fibers. Our Lady of Guadalupe's image provides all people with her love, compassion, help and protection. Many have her image as a tattoo to show their devotion to her. I was inspired to make this quilt upon seeing the tattoo depiction of Our Lady of Guadalupe on someone's arm. The shape and bright colors fascinated my artist eye.

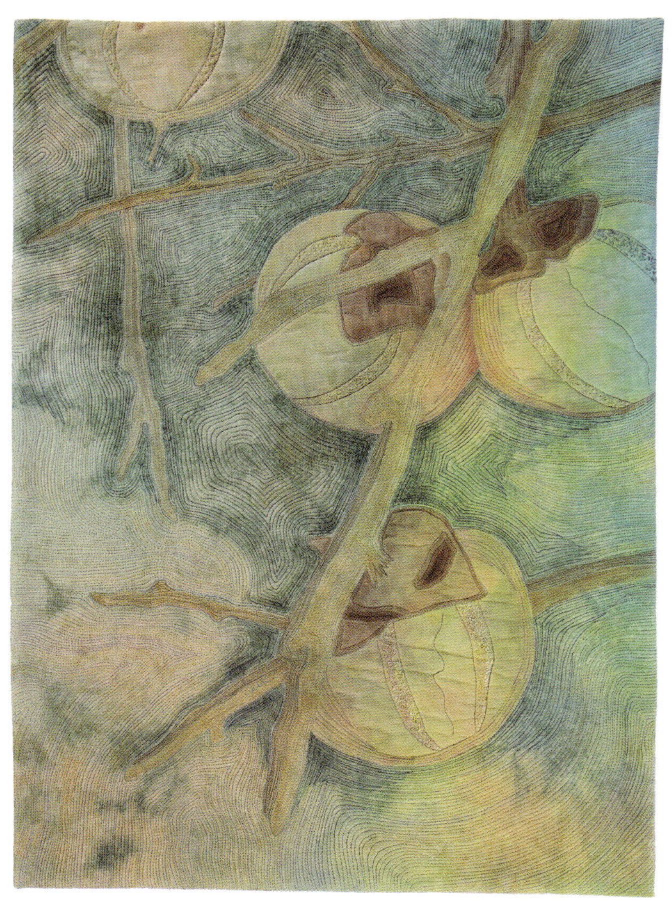

Nancy G Cook
Charlotte, NC, USA

Winter Fruit
28" x 38"

The persimmon fruit gives me inspiration for growing older. It is sweetest once touched with longer nights and a bit of frost, like people who grow sweeter and kinder with age.

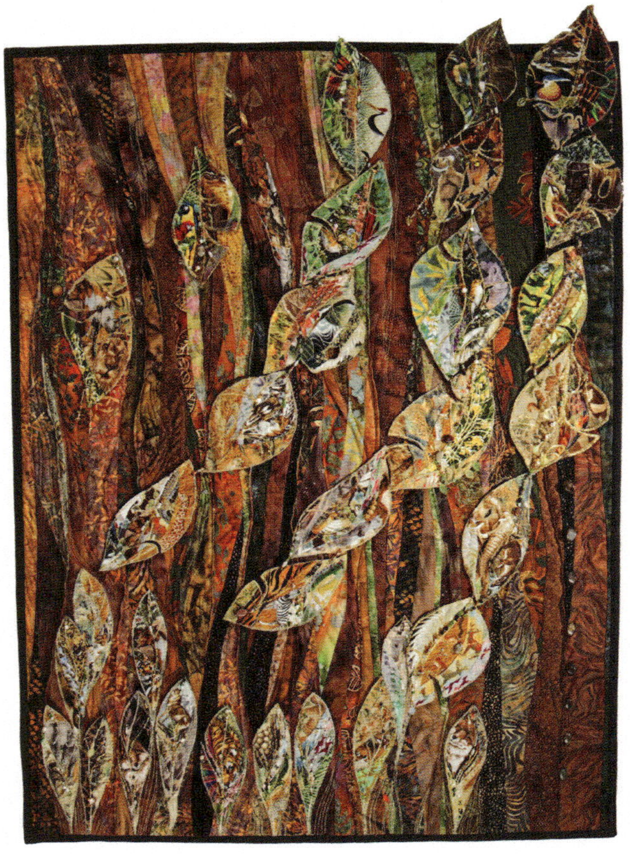

Peg Green
Reston, VA, USA

Shy Soul, Wild Soul
30" x 40"

This quilt was inspired by a sermon on self-discovery and finding inner courage. It was based on "A Hidden Wholeness" by Rev. Parker Palmer, describing our inner soul as "like a wild animal: tough, resilient, resourceful, savvy, and self-sufficient." ... Yet, like a wild animal, the soul is also shy; it seeks safety in the dense underbrush. I represented this idea with a dense forest background and all sorts of wild animals hidden in the leaves.

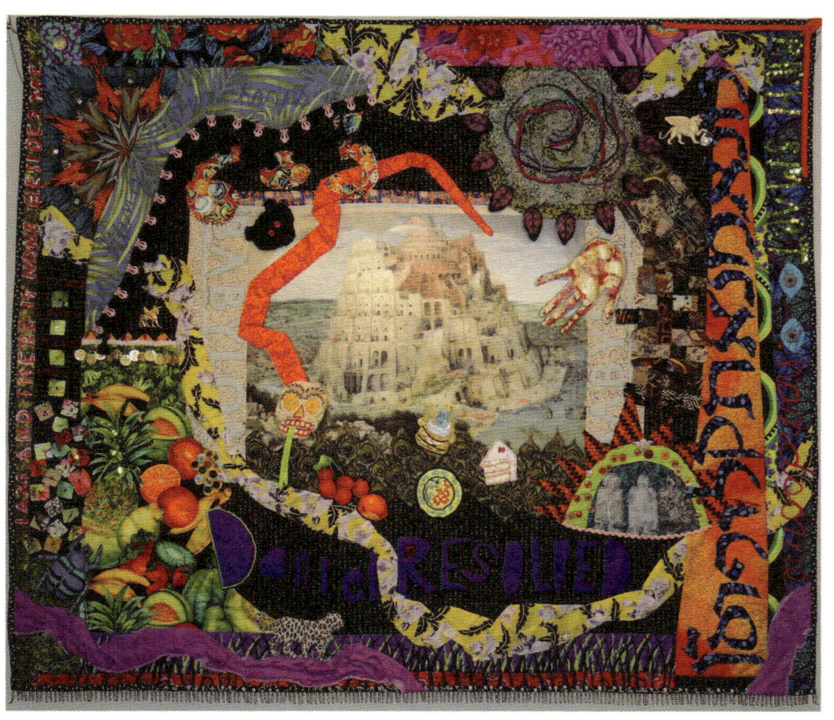

Kristy M Ottinger Greeneville, TN, USA

Off to Babylon or How I Spent My Summer Vacation, 605 B.C.
52" x 43"

Worship should originate from the heart of one's talents. Since I don't sing well, nor play an instrument, I began to art quilt as my own form of worship. Rather than sing notes of praise, I arranged colored fabric. As I began a study on the prophetic book of Daniel, I sewed my way through hours of meditation and prayer. This quilt was sewn after study of ancient Babylonian art and Daniel's prophetic writing. It was made as an act of worship to the God of Daniel.

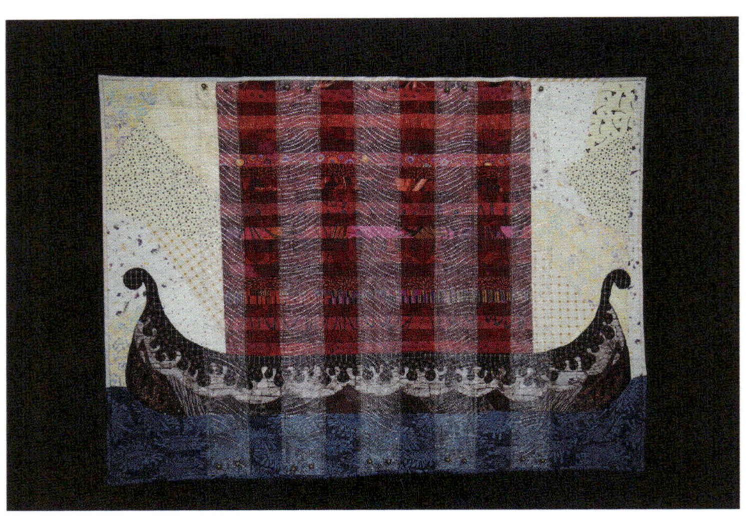

Ryn Pitts Fargo, ND, USA

Norway: My Journey to Northern Lights, Midsummer Nights
42" x 31"

The quilted Viking ship is a visual metaphor for my ancestors' journey to America in 1873. After visiting Stavanger harbor where they departed, I've longed for their stories--from the spellbinding beauty of Norwegian fjords to the harsh winters and unbroken Minnesota sod where they ultimately relocated. Genealogical research provided facts; family photos and letters offered more intimate details. The courage and perseverance they summoned to pursue the dream of a better life is now left to my imagination as I move along my ancestral journey a century and a half later.

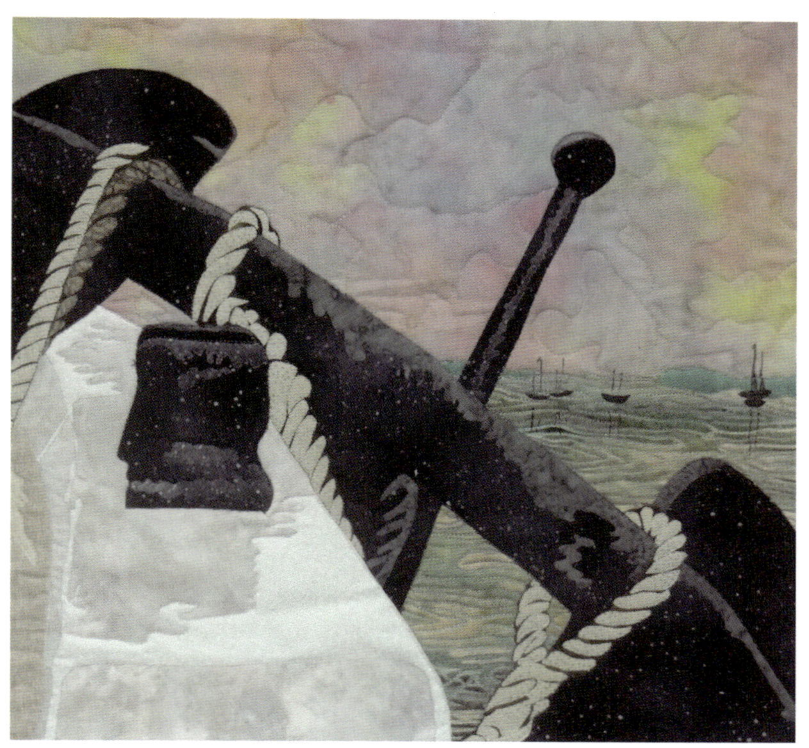

Stephanye Schuyler Portsmouth, NH, USA
After the Storm 22" x 20"

This fabric collage started as a photo I took on my summer vacation on the Maine schooner Victory Chimes. I am inspired by the majesty of these windjammers as well as the mercurial weather and beauty of Mid-Coast Maine.

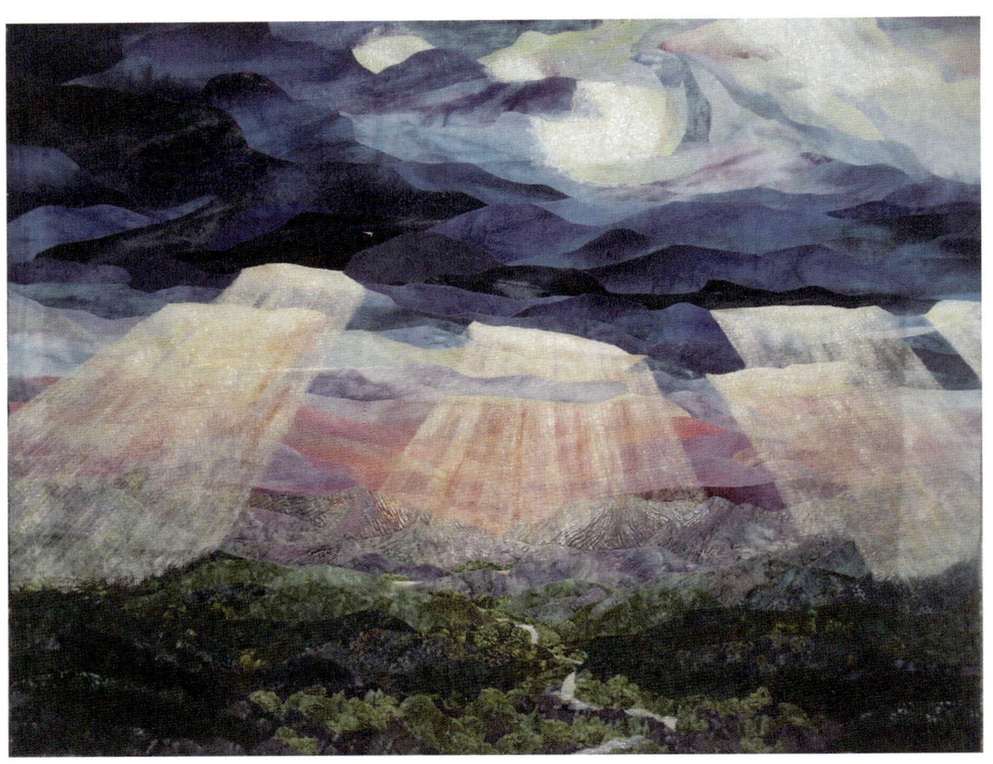

Linda S Schmidt Dublin, CA, USA
Benediction 87" x 65"

I have always loved the light, especially when it falls from heaven in golden beams after a thunderstorm. It's as if the Almighty was saying, "Some rain must fall to bring new life, but now be at peace, the storm is over; after the Darkness comes the Light." I took this picture from an airplane, following a frustrating 10-hour delay trying to get home. By the time we left, I was a frustrated mess, but when I looked out the window and saw this scene, it was worth it just to see this beauty, and my cares fell away.

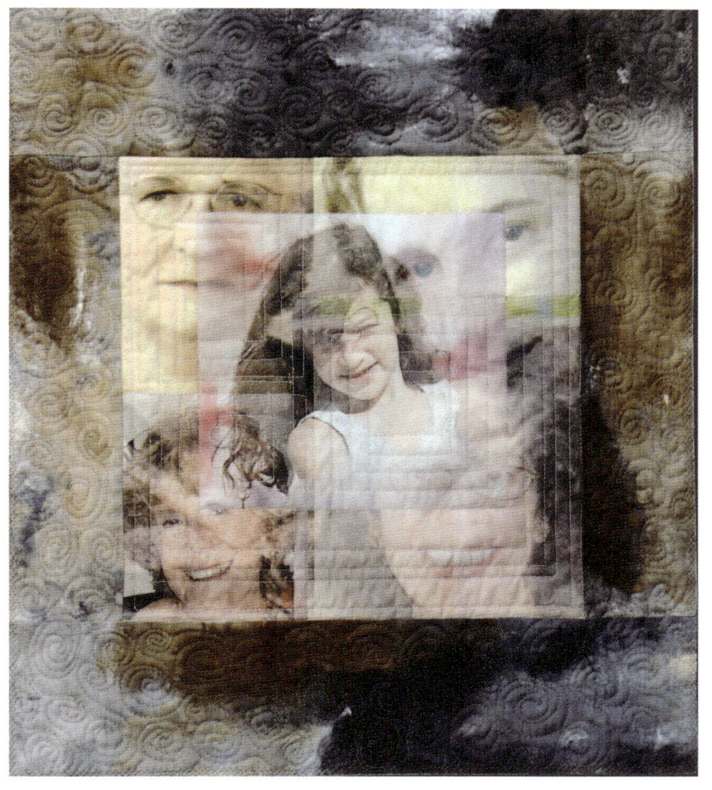

Bonnie D Askowitz Miami, FL, USA

"L'dor V'dor (From Generation to Generation)"
18.25" x 20.25"

This quilt is a self portrait and family biography depicting five generations of women from my family. We are bound by bloodlines, culture, religion, and nationality making us one. At the same time, we are influenced by the eras in which we live, making us distinctly different. We continue to make our marks on the world.

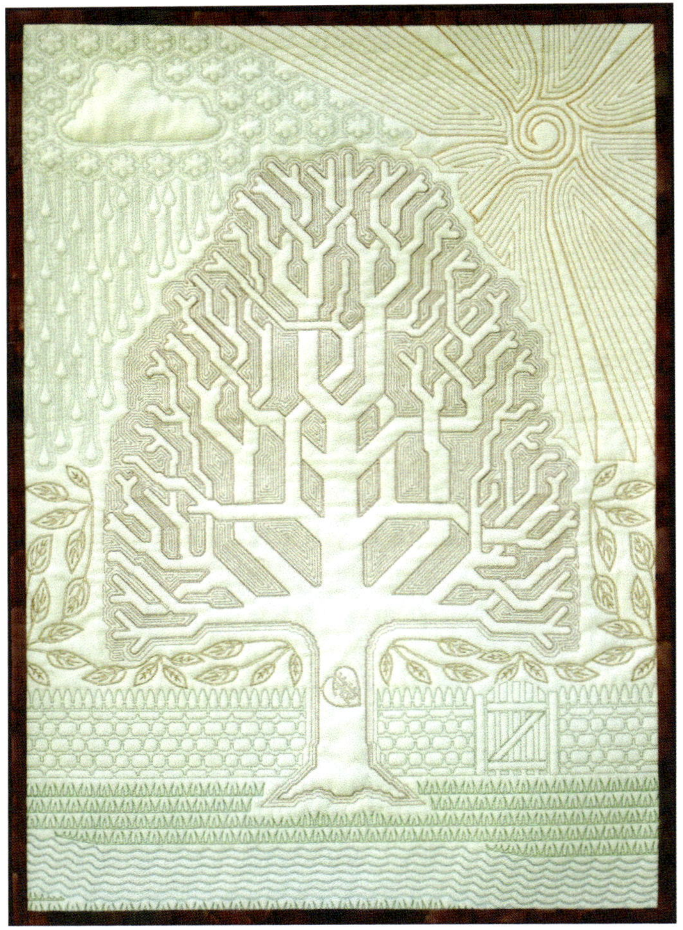

Albert Feldman
Rockville, MD, USA

A Tribute to Kilmer"
19" x 26"

The beauty and majesty of nature, and trees in particular, have provided inspiration to many people. This quilt had two sources of inspiration. The primary inspiration was the poem "Trees" by Joyce Kilmer. The inspiration for the tree itself came from a large tree with maroon leaves that I had seen as a youth in the Bronx's Van Cortlandt Park. My wife and I used to walk near this tree when we were engaged in 1959, so I included a heart inscribed with our initials. Besides the tree, other elements in the quilt are leaves, the sun, rain, snow, a cloud, a gated stone fence, a stream, and grass.

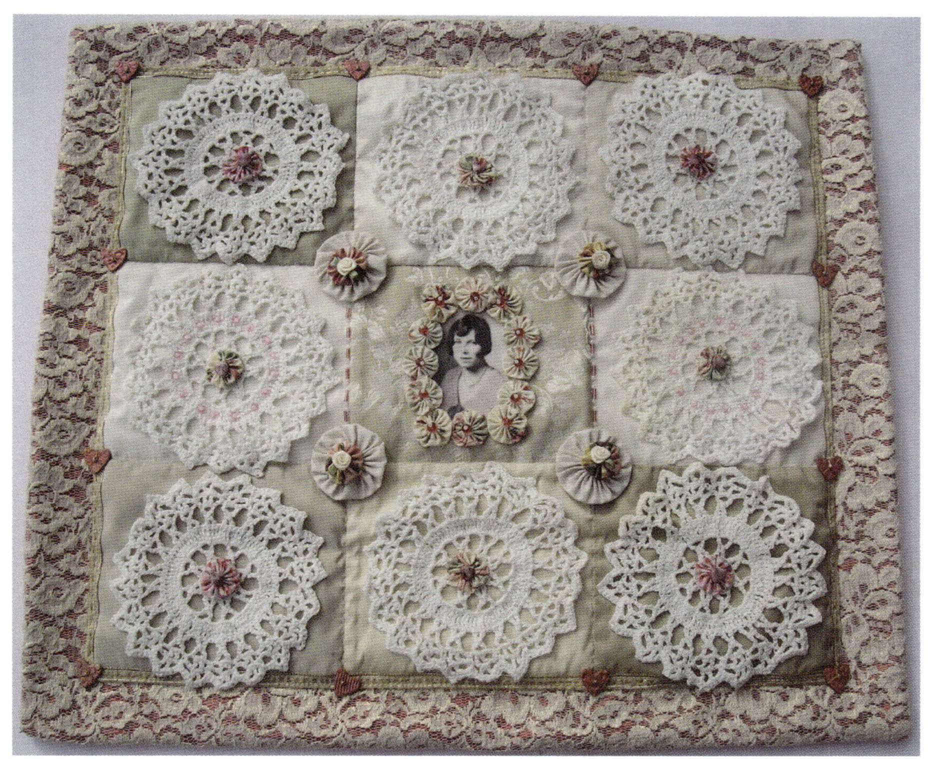

Marcia Tuznik West Chester, OH, USA
The Aunt Ruth Quilt 22" x 19"

My Aunt Ruth was a wonderful woman who lived to be 96 years old. I have fond memories of visiting Aunt Ruth and learning to crochet and cross-stitch. Aunt Ruth really knew how to live. She went to Mass every morning and had a stiff drink every evening. Aunt Ruth had a lot of energy and her hands were always busy crocheting something: doilies for tablecloths or coasters, hats, scarves, afghans, poodles to hide your toilet paper. After her death I came across these coaster doilies. Although some have coffee stains on them, they remind me of her great legacy.

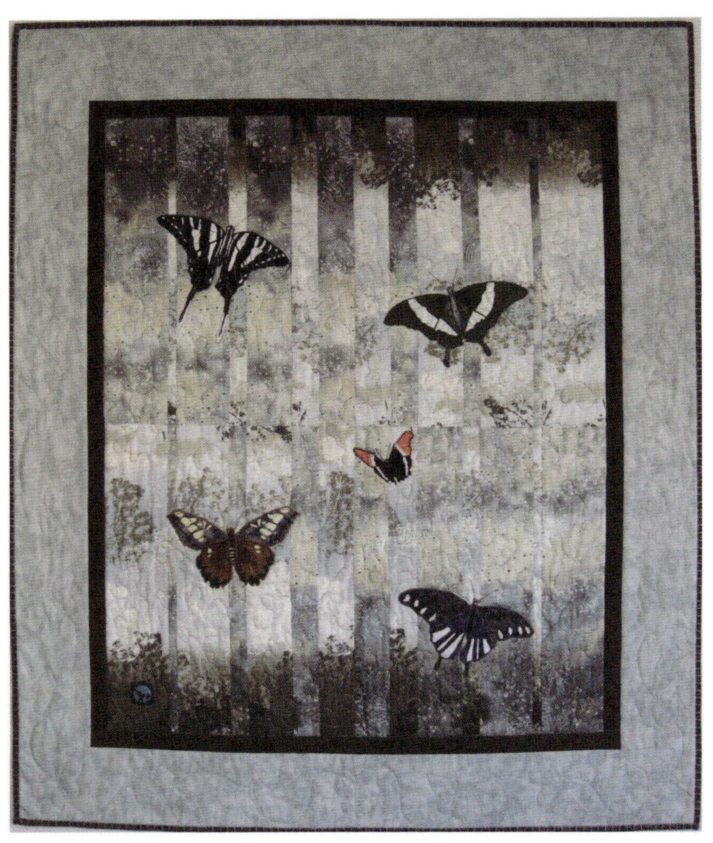

Barbara Dahlberg Crofton, MD, USA
Flight 38" x 44"

I have long been fascinated with butterflies, their beauty and delicacy, their wondrous change from caterpillars to flowers in flight. The butterfly has become my personal symbol of transformation and liberation. Flight is my expression of joyful breaking free of restriction to grow creatively, throw away doubts and fly as an artist.

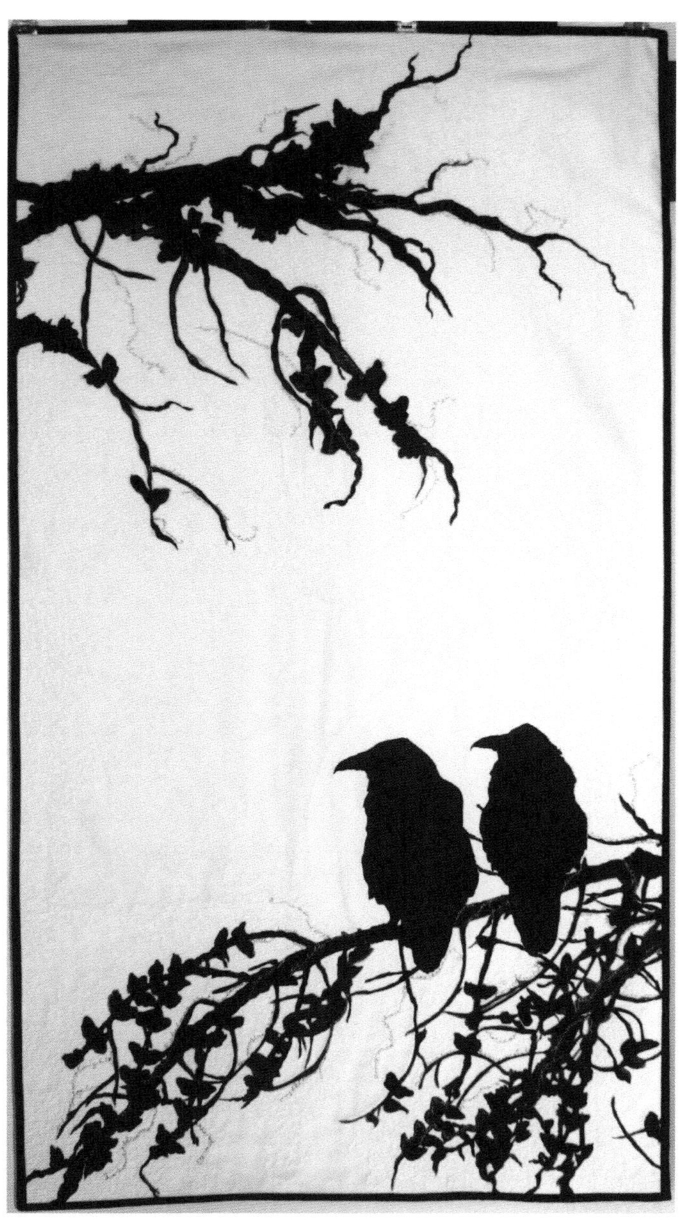

Stacy Hurt
Orange, CA, USA

Moon Sisters
30” x 53”

I was so inspired by Sting's song 'Sister Moon' that I painted these Ravens sitting atop a tree in front of the moon enjoying the lyrical and floating melody. I believe Ravens to be one of my spirit guides.

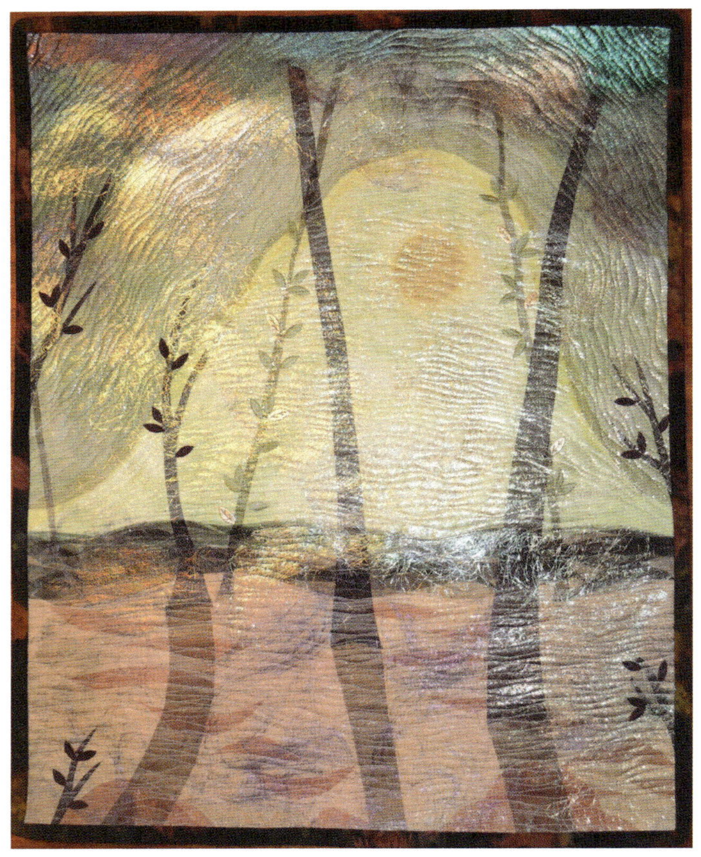

Dabney H Narvaez
Reston, VA, USA

Sunrise at the Cabin 20" x 24"

We all need a place, imagined or real, where we can go for solace and inspiration. My place is a small, wooded property in Sullivan County, N.Y., nestled in the foothills of the Catskill Mountains. I have gone there ever since my husband and I were married forty-three years ago. I have rejoiced there, wept there, found comfort and inner strength. The design for this quilt is based on a photo I took on a recent visit. It was early morning and the sun was filtering through the trees. As with life's journey, light and shadow intermingle. It was a moment of gentle and restorative peace.

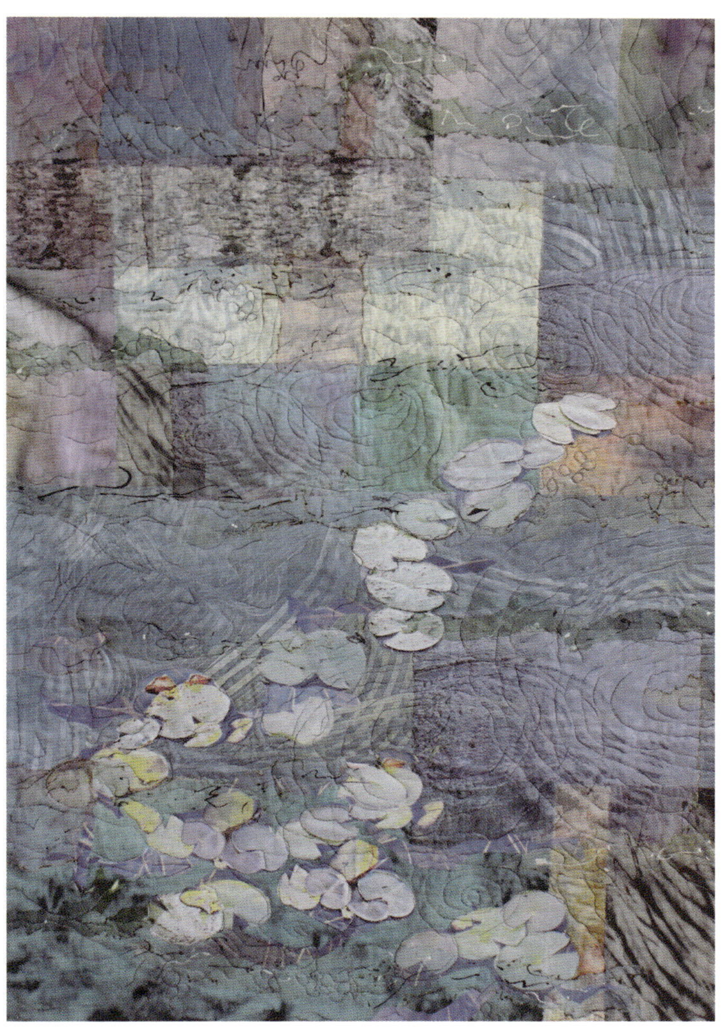

Annette Rogers
Raleigh, NC, USA

Peaceful Waters
26" x 36"

Water has always been a meaningful symbol to me. I find comfort and peace in the rushing sound of a waterfall, in the babbling of a brook, and in the quiet surroundings of a pond. In difficult times, and in times of praise and thanksgiving, water refreshes me.

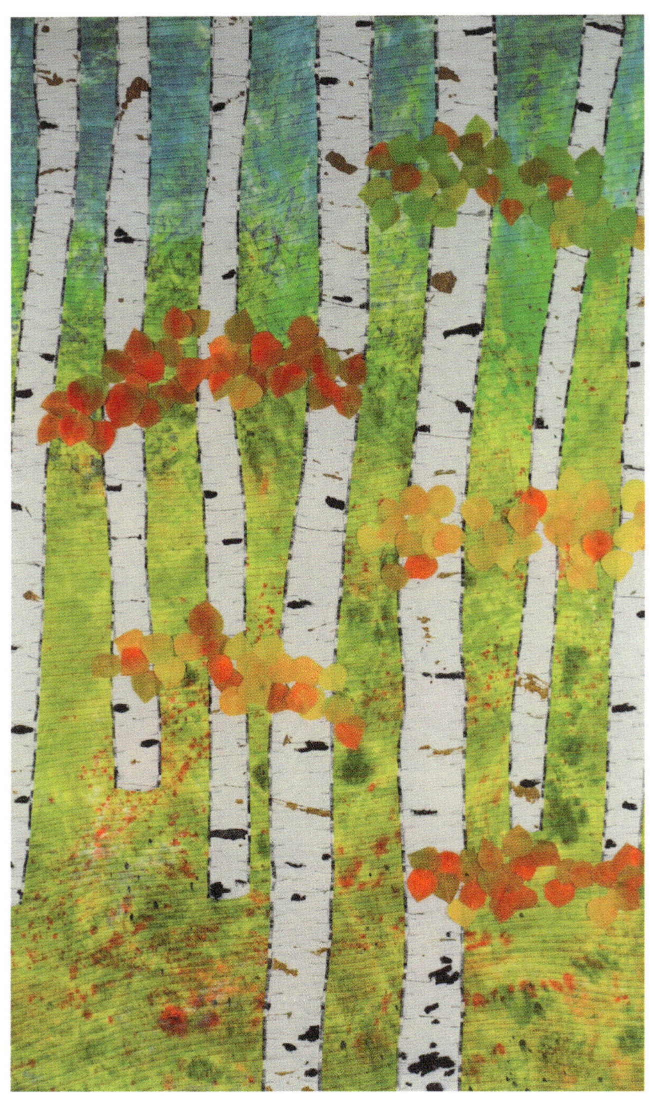

Gerrie Congdon
Portland, OR, USA

High Desert Aspen Grove 42" x 52"

I get excited when I see a grove of Aspens. I love the way they grow in clumps from a mother tree. The trunks are generally long and slender and marked by thick black horizontal scars and prominent black knots. It looks as if someone walked through the grove with a paint brush and drew lines and black dabs on each trunk. The leaves, a beautiful rounded shape, change color from green to yellow, orange and red in the fall. They are often called quaking Aspens because the leaves rustle in the wind. Using natural beauty in my art adds a spiritual dimension to my creativity.

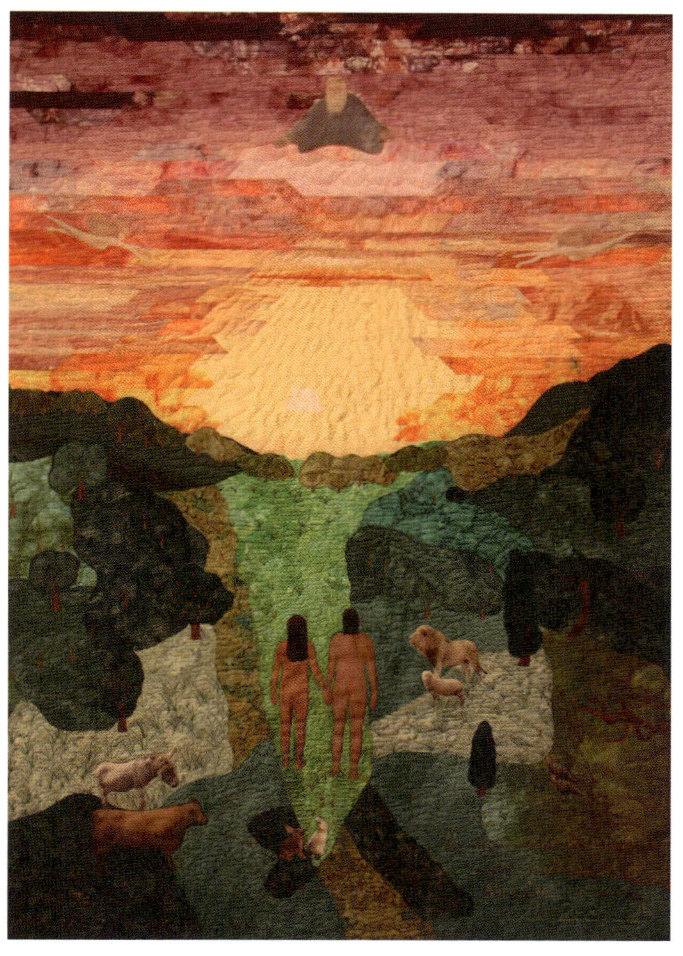

Frances Krupka
Traverse City, MI, USA

Original Innocence: The Wedding of Adam and Eve
39.5" x 52.75"

The magnificence of creation comes to a peak in Genesis 2:24-25 as God gives us the gift of marriage. In these words describing the world before the Fall we find perfect tranquility. Man and woman exist in perfect innocence. This second account of creation serves as the platform for our ministry to couples preparing for marriage. We encourage them to bring to their marriage part of Eden in its perfection. This quilted image was made to capture the joy, wonder and innocence that are possible in marriage. May it bring joy to all who see it.

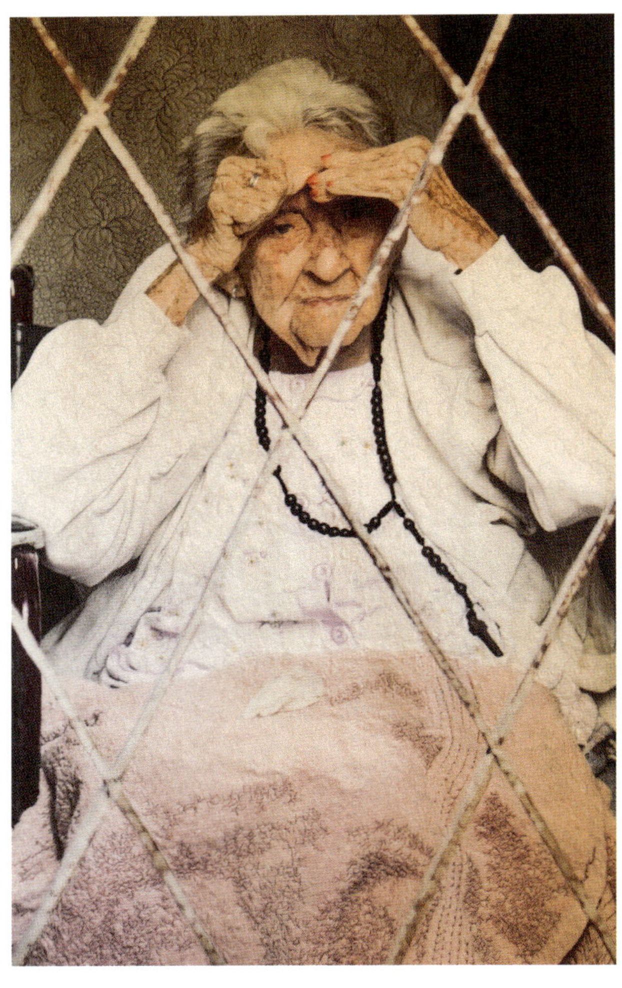

Jennifer Day
Santa Fe, NM, USA

Memories
31" x 45"

This is the image of a ninety-six year old woman sitting in her wheelchair in her doorway in Havana, Cuba. She is wearing jewelry, her hair is brushed and her nails are polished. I love that she still has memories of her husband and that her wedding ring now rests on her right hand. She's staring out the door, perhaps remembering her life during the glory days of Havana in the 1950's,when she was in the prime of her life. Her face, hands,hair and the doorway bars are 100% covered in thread, the rest is free motion embroidery.

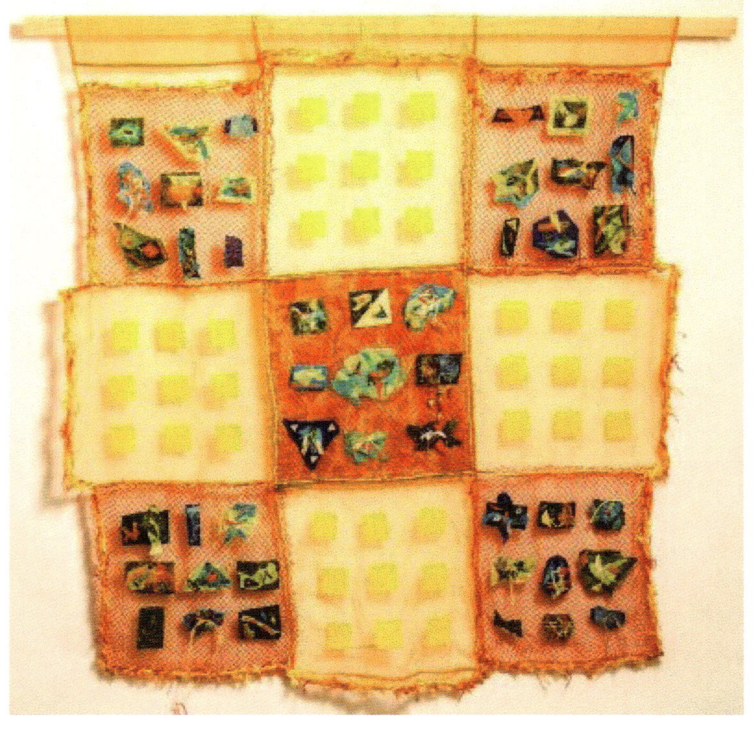

Connie Conrad
Atlanta, GA, USA

Redemption
48" x 48"

"Redemption" renders what was once considered insignificant or no longer useful into something of value, of beauty or of renewed purpose. In this "scrappy 9-patch" quilt, the too-small scraps, cast off packaging and other discards have been resurrected together as a thing of beauty and grace. By bringing the individual pieces together, what could not survive alone is transformed into a representation of what we are inspired to know through faith, that "redemption" is our promise and our reality. We see this redemption taking place; we help it along in ourselves and others; and with God's grace, it is our ultimate resting place.

Kasia O
Delafield, WI, USA

Transformation
36" x 36"

When we walk the labyrinth of Life, transformation often occurs. Starting with the idea of life's changes, the word "Transformation" was made into a circular (mandala) stencil that was painted onto the background fabric. Next, rays of transformational light were painted into place. The piece was quilted and the cording attached in a labyrinth fashion to suggest the journey from here to THERE. A crystal placed in the center represents our soul - the LIGHT within. Mandalas are my fascination. I create personalized LoveLights©, with hidden messages or names worked into the design for the JOY of the recipient.

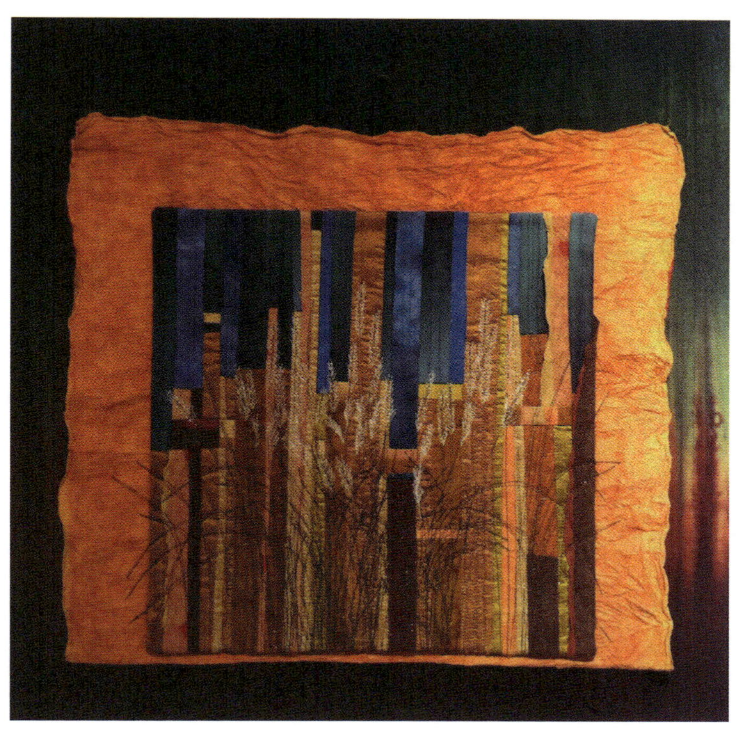

Joan Bratton Woodridge, IL, USA

Autumn Grasses 21" x 20"

Frequent walks with friends in the Questor's group inspired this piece. The group meets early mornings twice a week to walk the trails of the Morton Arboretum. It feeds the soul and spirit to walk with friends in faith and appreciate the changing richness of the landscape throughout the seasons. Autumn prairie grasses highlighted against the backdrop of a Midwestern blue sky are depicted using threadwork and natural fibers.

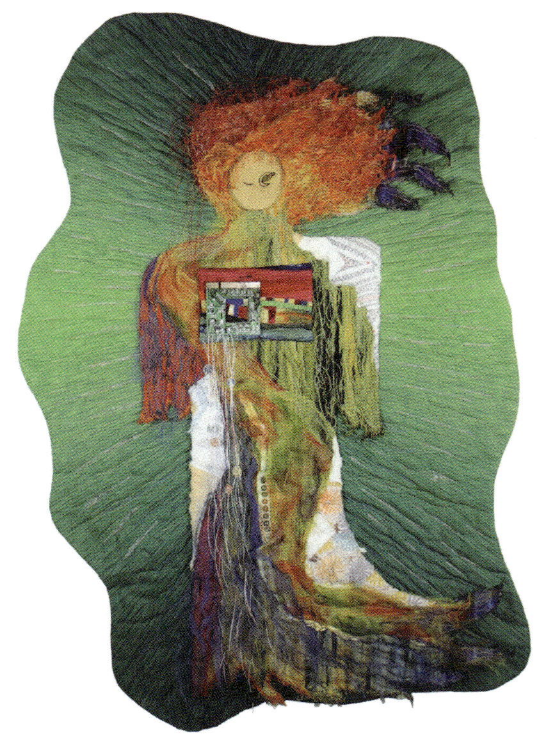

Helen Brisson
Bend, OR, USA

Spirit Within
24” x 33”

"Spirit Within" was created for a juried show through the Arts, Beautification and Culture Commission in Bend, Oregon. The theme was "Inside Out", how Bend's external environment inspires our internal environment (mental, physical, emotional and spiritual.)

"Spirit Within" uses objects that might be seen as ugly or useless. All of the integrated items have a personality, and a history that when uniquely considered can take the observer away from simply seeing a work of art. Did the scrapes of fabric once enfold a loved one? Did the foil protect an offering for a crying child? Did the computer board allow a homebound person to communicate with the world?

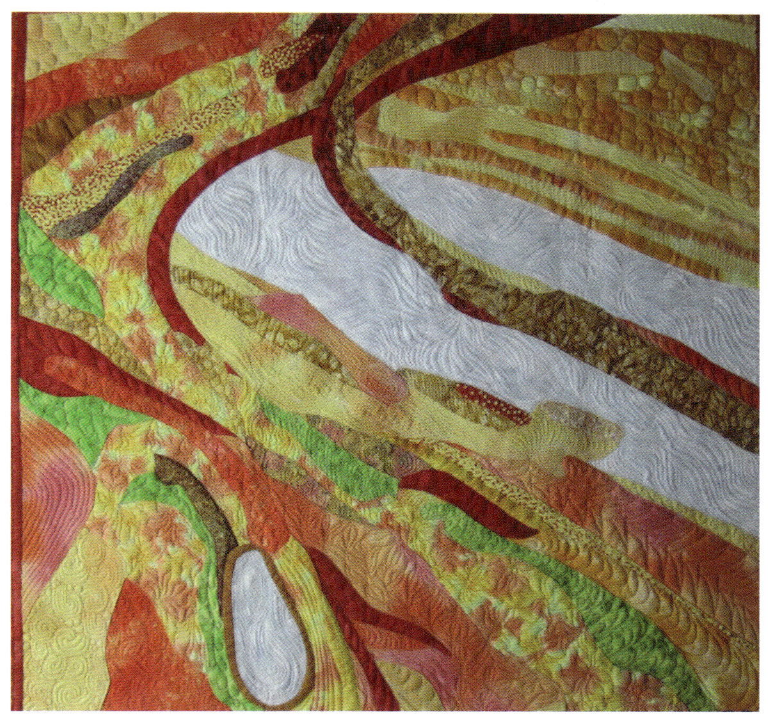

Julia F Gaff
Lusby, MD, USA

The Flow
34" x 33.5"

Like life, "The Flow", just happened. In October I paid $2 for a used book -- "Design Explorations for the Creative Quilter" by Katie Pasquini Masopust. This led to trying Katie's Blind Painting on Thanksgiving Day. Using her techniques, I cautiously completed "The Flow", thrilled as an expression of myself unfolded. Art Quilters, sponsored by Cyndi Souder, gave me the assurance to complete "The Flow".

While quilting, I wondered what this really is - water, music, the American West, sexuality, life unto death back into life. "The Flow" is all of these. It represents the essence of being connected.

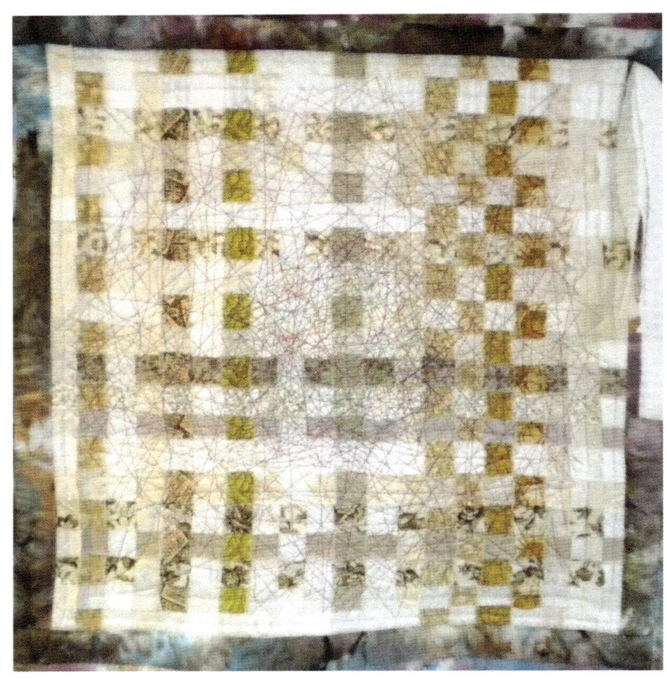

Dianne D Bullach
Arlington, VA, USA

[RE]MIX
26" x 26"

As a youth mission chaperone, my job included planning a closing devotion using the camp themes [RE]MIX: [re]think, [re]do, [re]create, [re]act. Making a quilt came to mind, so on the bus trip, everyone tore a 1-inch strip from my stash, then brought it to our final meeting to place on the batting.

While quilting I wrote:

"Like fabric, we start out whole, smooth, bright, new, unique.

We become torn, frayed, isolated, lost, soiled, knotted, creased, and wrinkled.

God selects us, touches us, presses us, backs us up, and weaves us together.

His WORD is embroidered on our hearts.

We become part of a greater whole, textured, brighter, stronger, warmer, more useful."

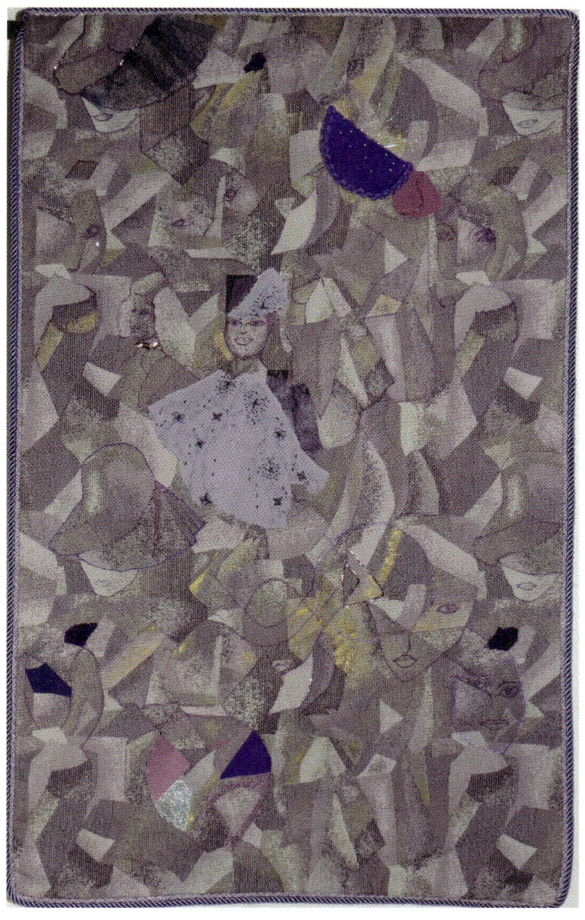

Pat Johnson
Durham, NC, USA

Faces
32” x 52.5”

This quilt is dedicated to and celebrates the many faces of women.

Tapestries are beautifully mysterious and complex. Just as a sculptor sees an art image in a piece of marble, I began to see faces in this tapestry. In fact, the more I studied the more faces began to reveal themselves. Some were full faces, others only fragments, like a mardi gras mask. It reminded me of the many faces we as women wear.The techniques used to highlight the women include hand embroidery, beading, needle punch, felting, painting and quilting.

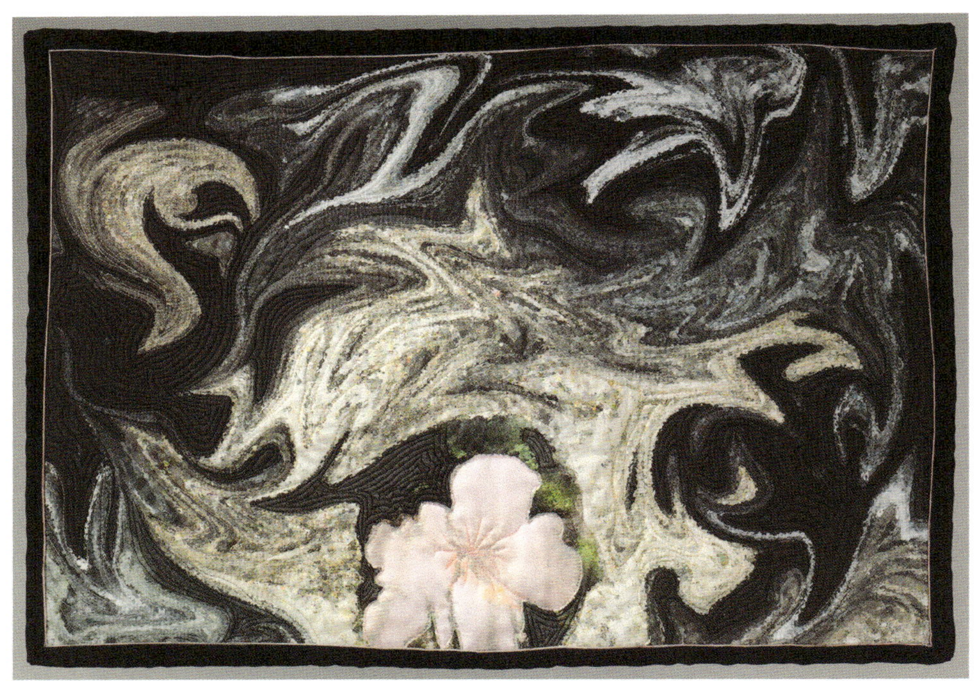

Judy Warner
Victor, NY, USA
Emergence 25.5" x 17.5"

In the darkest of moments and most confusing of times, the flower in this art quilt reminds me to look for the positive and know the power of that choice. By choosing love and healing, we can bring light and hope to even the most tragic of settings. We can be inspiration.

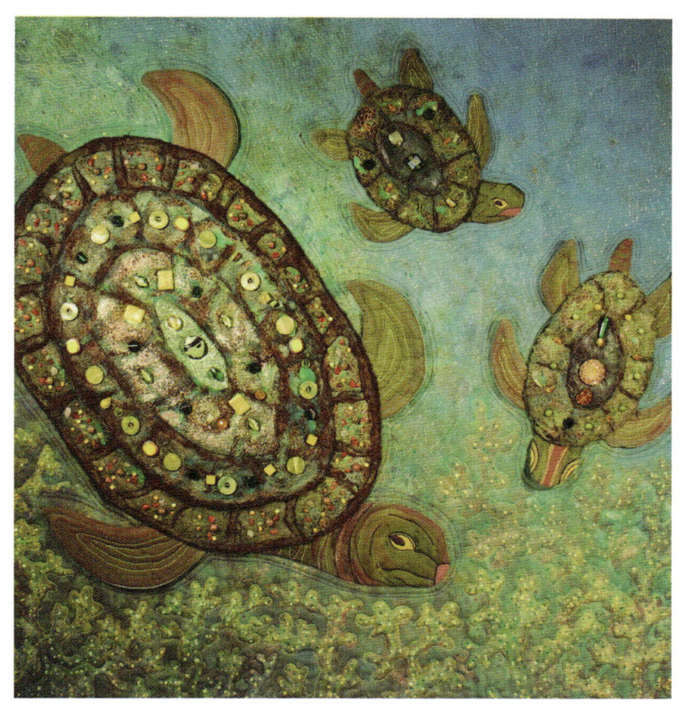

Barb Forrister
Austin, TX, USA

Emerald Treasures
33" x 31"

"Emerald Treasures" is an inspirational touchstone piece for me. After it was created, it left immediately for a show. On its way home, it was caught in a conveyor belt and the large turtle head was completely decapitated and a large piece of her shell was missing. I was devastated, especially after receiving notice that it was accepted into IQF West Coast Wonders special exhibit. It sat on my table for a couple of weeks because I didn't know what to do. Finally, I had to try and fix the piece in hopes that she might travel once again. I had no idea how to do this or if it could even be done. I repainted another head and attached it. Luckily, I still had beads and leftover materials that matched for rebuilding her shell.. There were holes that went through the entire quilt. Mistyfuse and fused fabric covered these area. Finally, she seemed ready to travel and make her way to Festival where she was featured in the program. Emerald Treasures has been an inspiration to me to never give up even when presented with adverse situations; hope prevails.

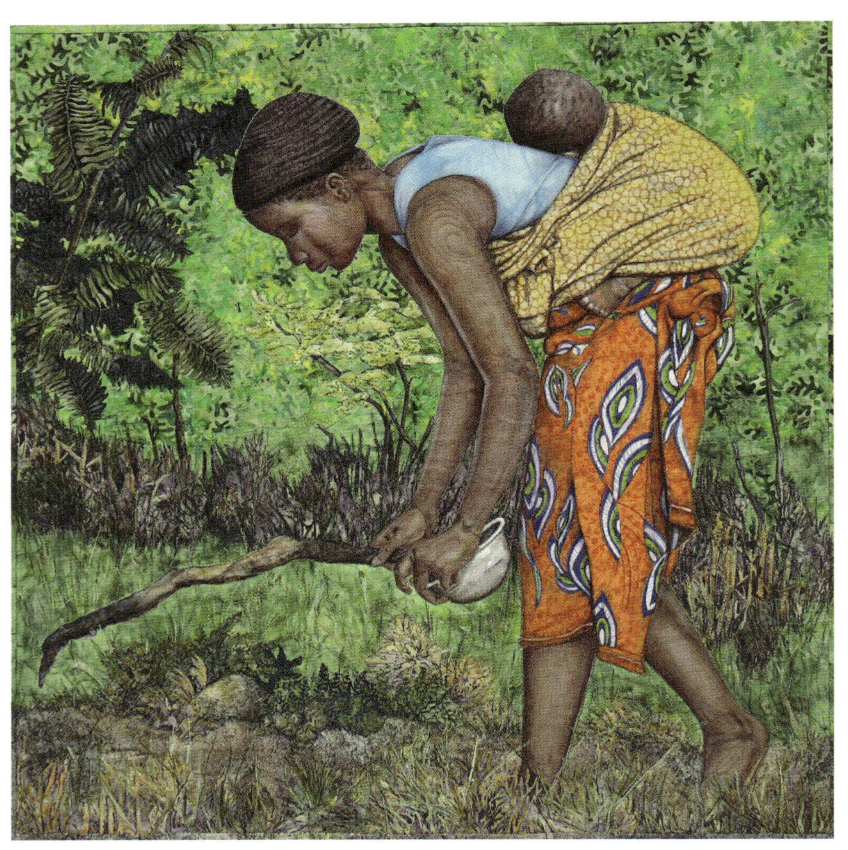

Cherrie Hampton Oklahoma City, OK, USA
Cultivator 30" x 31"

Images of women involved in their arduous daily activities have impressed me with the difficulty of life for most of the rest of the world. These women go about the daunting tasks of carrying water, tending children and planting gardens with a determined strength of body and mind that can be lost in the midst of a fast paced mechanized society.

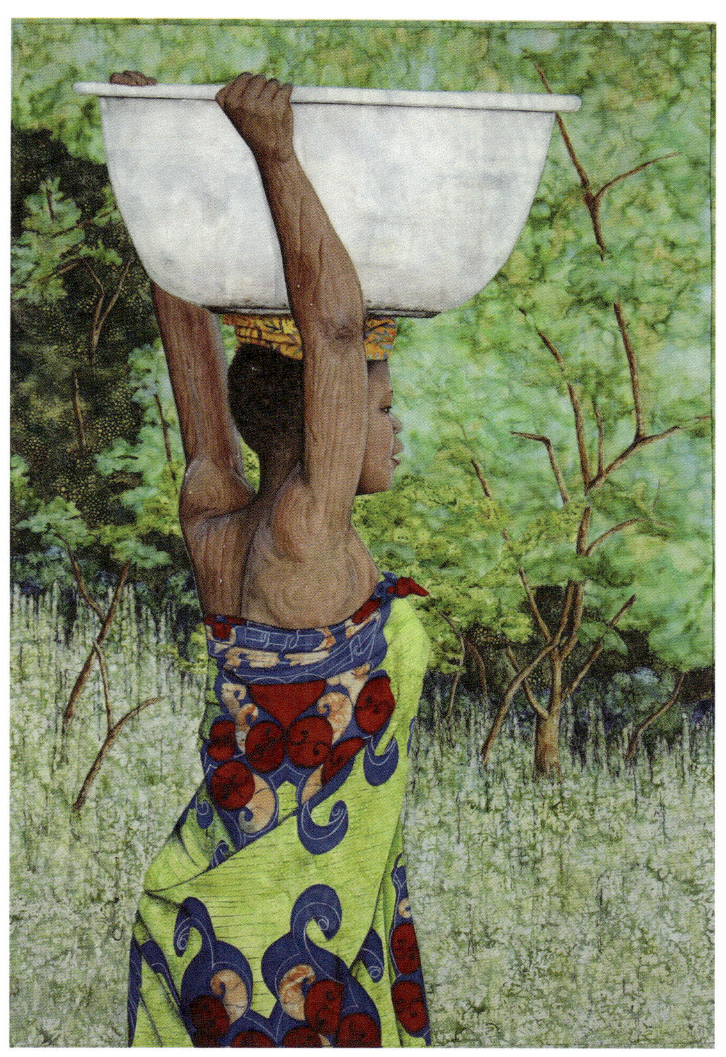

Cherrie Hampton
Oklahoma City,
OK, USA

Waterbearer
30" x 43"

As I worked on these quilts my heart was inspired with a new compassion for the daily struggles of those around me.

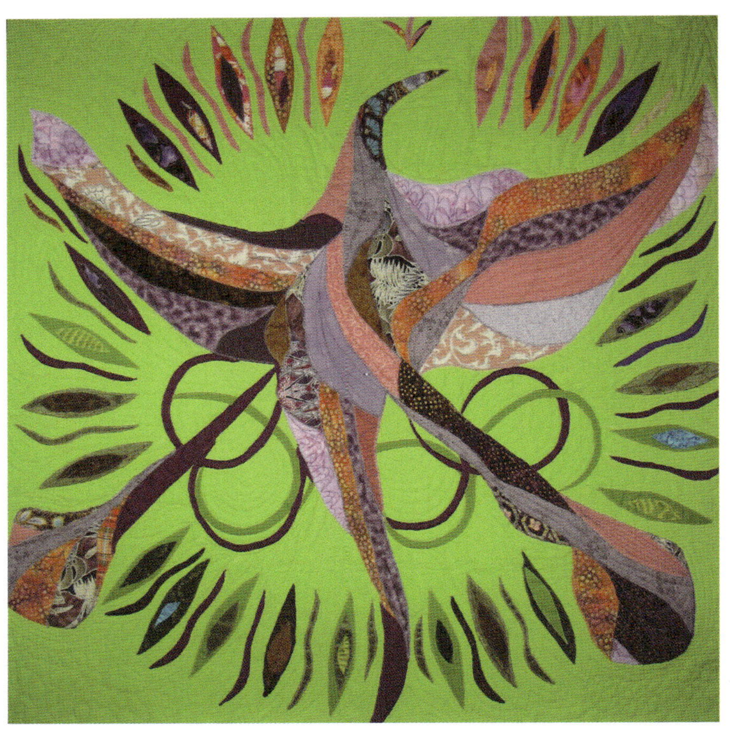

Kathleen Turner Tallahassee, FL, USA
Hope 35" x 35"

At a time when I was nearly out of hope, a dried-up orchid blossom pinned to my design wall called to me. It had lost color and beauty, but I sketched and pieced it anyway. Surprising beauty emerged - part flower, part mandala, part firebird. Hope.

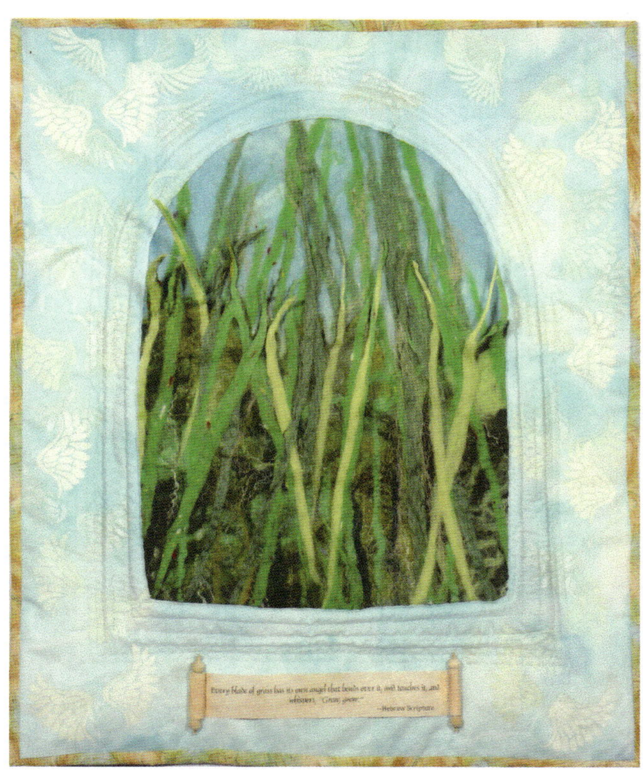

Diane L Cadrain
West Hartford, CT, USA

Every Blade of Grass has its Own Angel
26" x 29"

As a Catholic/Unitarian mother of a cantor in the Jewish faith, mother-in-law of a rabbi, and wife of a man raised as a Jew, I have come to know and appreciate words of great beauty and comfort in Jewish spiritual writings. This statement, originating in a text called the Midrash, a commentary on the Hebrew Bible, came to me through The Artist's Way by Julia Cameron, a book encouraging artists to honor their spirits, which has been a powerful catalyst in my sacred journey as an artist.

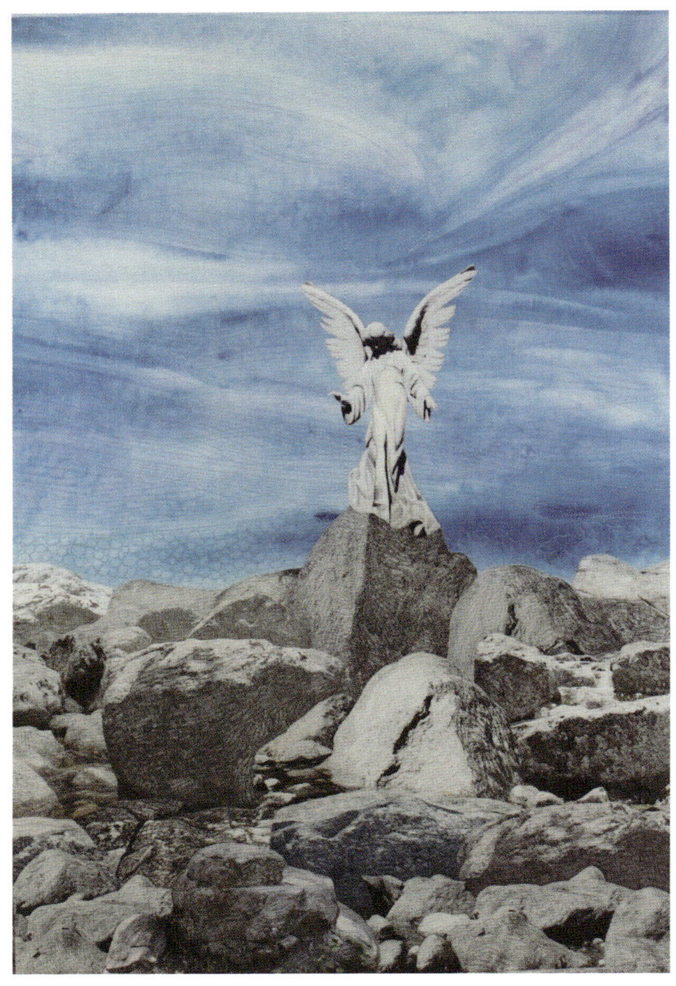

Joanna Monroe
Hudson Falls, NY, USA

Interlude
24" x 34"

The forests and mountains are my retreat and spending time in the woods provides me with solitude and nurtures my creativity. I often feel that if I could turn quickly enough I will see my guardian angel, a constant and almost tangible presence, beside me as I roam the trails and summit the peaks. I am thankful to have my guardian angel to accompany me on my journey.

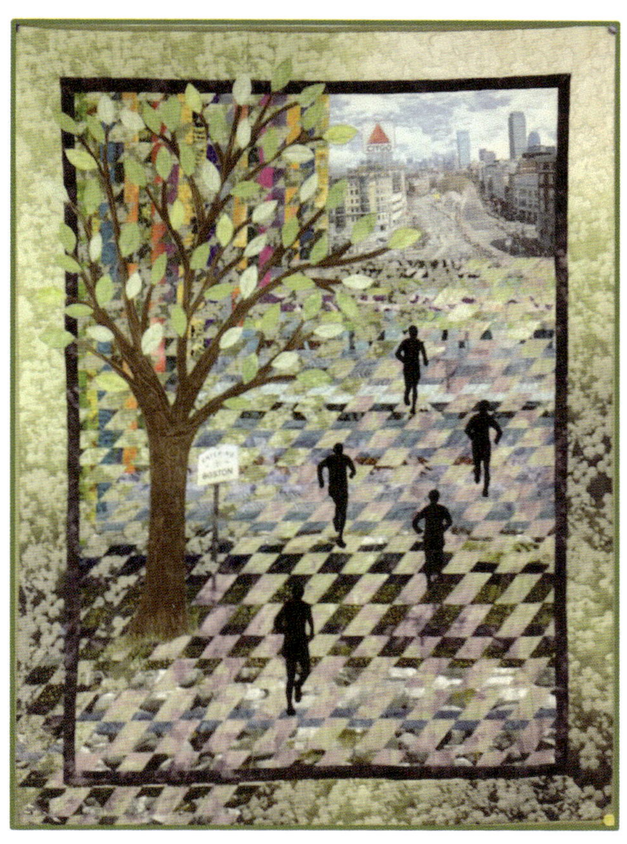

Rosanne F Williamson
Warrenton, VA, USA

Boston in the Spring
30.5" x 40"

Five times in the spring, I traveled to New England to support my husband as he ran the 26.2 miles of the prestigious Boston Marathon. The strength and commitment of the runners, the beauty of the city, and the pride I feel in my husband as he races inspired this quilt and my desire to challenge myself as a quilt artist. "But they that wait upon the LORD shall renew their strength; they shall mount up with wings as eagles; they shall run, and not be weary; and they shall walk, and not faint." Isaiah 40:31

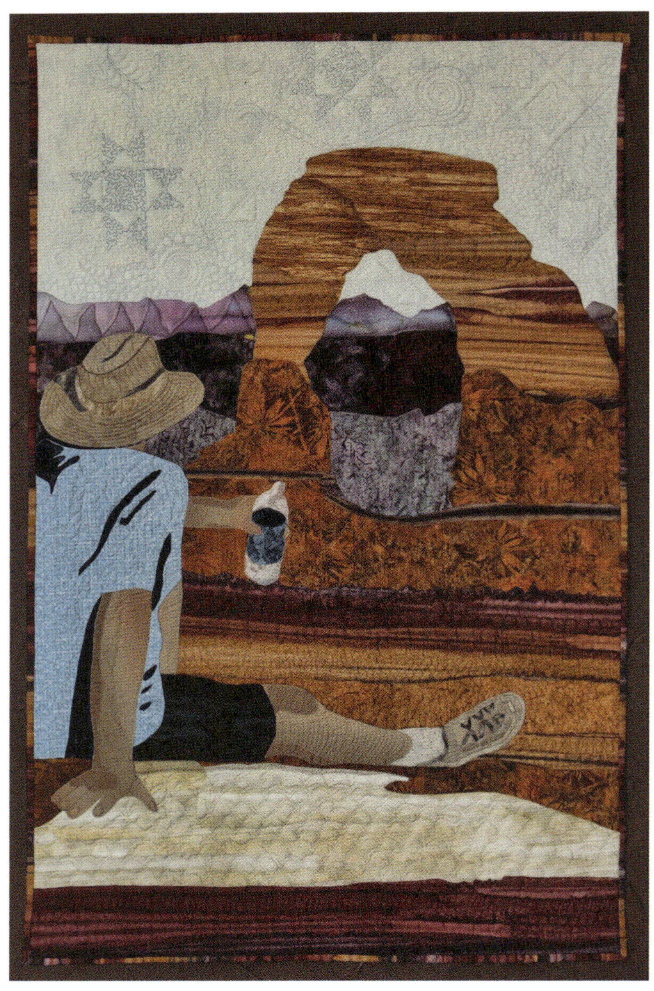

Marj Luchtenburg
Waukee, LA, USA

Moab, Utah
30" x 45"

Canyonlands National Park, near Moab, Utah, contains dozens of red sandstone arches carved by wind erosion over eons. At the Delicate Arch I took this photo of my husband. The park is one of God's most grand and reverent sanctuaries. How many people and animals have gazed upon these magnificent structures before my time? The hike brought to mind Psalm 90:4 – "For a thousand years in your sight are like a day that has just gone by, or like a watch in the night." I acknowledge that I feel important to God as one of his loved creations, yet sometimes I feel very small.

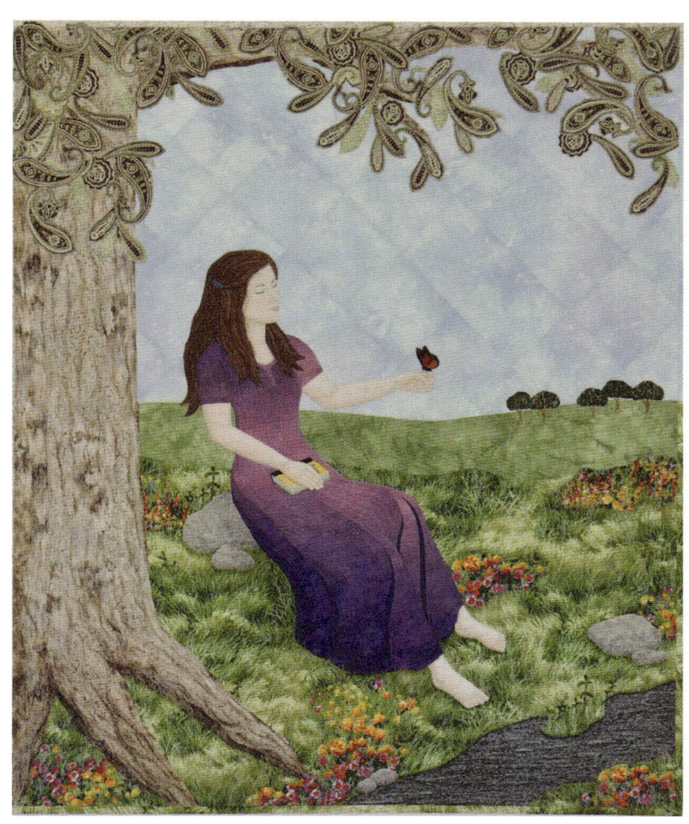

Sharon L Schlotzhauer
Colorado Springs, CO USA

He Leads Me By Still Waters
36.5" x 42"

The book of Psalms is very inspirational and one of my favorite books in the Bible. When I feel joy or sorrow; when I'm distressed or sad and need comfort; or when I want to read words of praise and worship this is where I turn. The 23rd Psalm is special to me personally because the LORD is my Shepherd. This quilt portrays the gentle beauty and peace of resting by His "still" or "quiet" waters. The large, strong tree can represent God and the "shade" He is for His children.

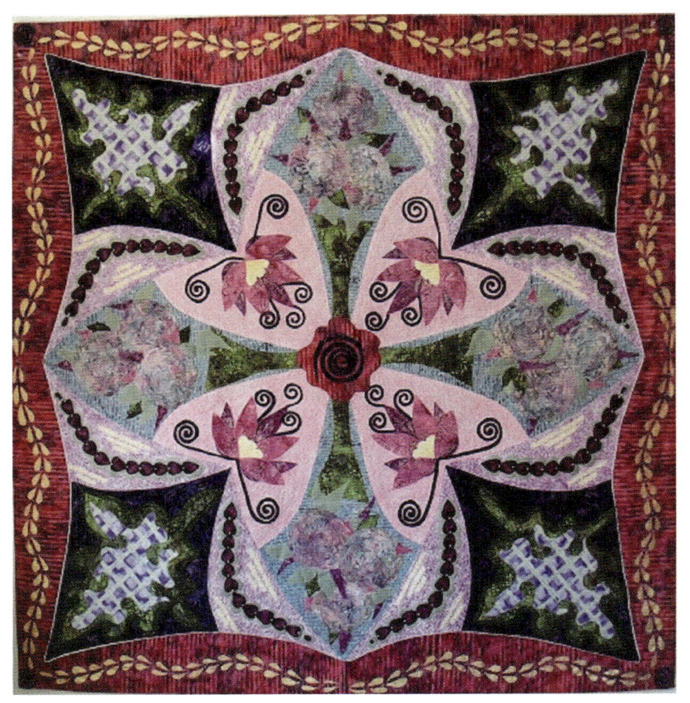

Christine Somerset
Tucson, AZ, USA

Crossroads
51.5" x 52"

"Crossroads" expresses the inspiration I receive when opposites meet. In my life, the work-world met retirement, belonging met newness, the Northwest met the Southwest. Where opposites meet there is always challenge, experimentation, problem resolution, and new opportunities. In my quilting I am especially interested in expressing a flow of energy that tells a story. In "Crossroads" my core self is represented by the spiral center. The pink energy flows toward the center while the green energy flows outward. I am fed, and I give back. This is my source of inspiration.

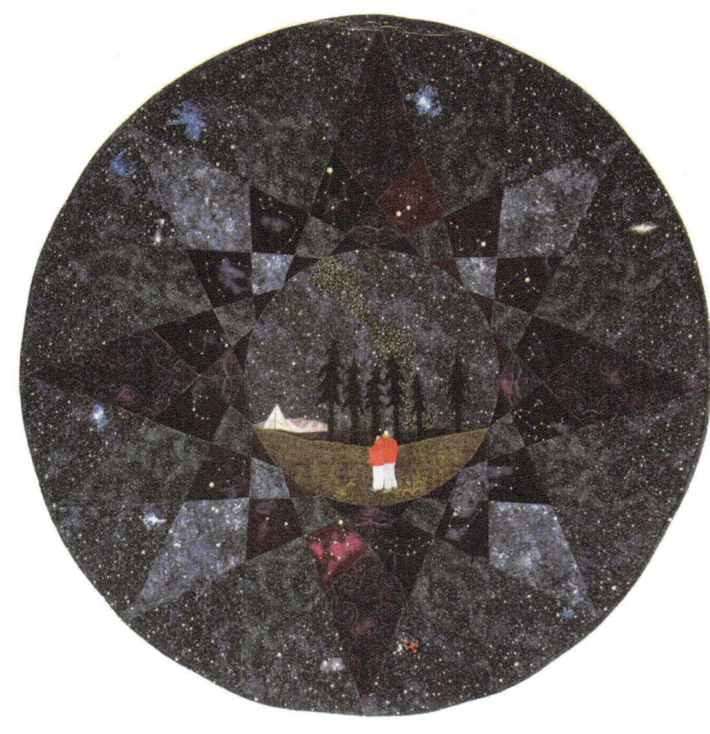

Alice M Magorian
Catonsville, MD, USA

Celestial Navigation 48" x 48"

This quilt is for my husband, Dan, whose sense of adventure and vision, of being at home in a large universe have enabled me to go places and experience things I would never have on my own. It is also inspired by the way a very ordinary experience can turn on a dime and suddenly become a glimpse of something both luminous and limitless.

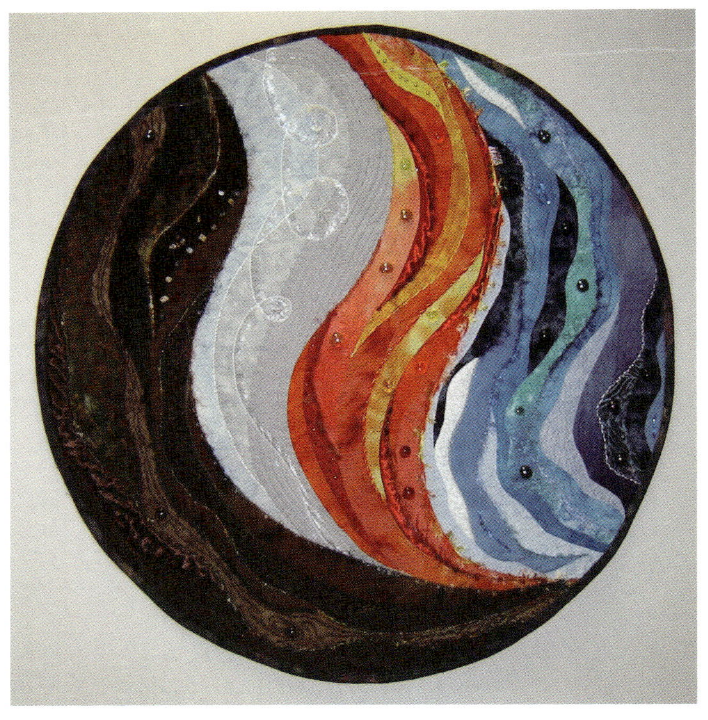

Angela J Maves
Pembroke,
Ontario, Canada

Elementals--
Earth Spirits
30" x 30"

I created this wall quilt for an Earth Day Celebration. Each invited artist was asked to create a piece to represent the earth and what is meant to them. When I thought about the four elements, Earth, Wind, Fire and Water, I wanted to show the light and dark, positive and negative, life giving and life destroying nature of each and how each force is balanced in the spinning of our world. Each element spirals and twists in our earthly dance of life.

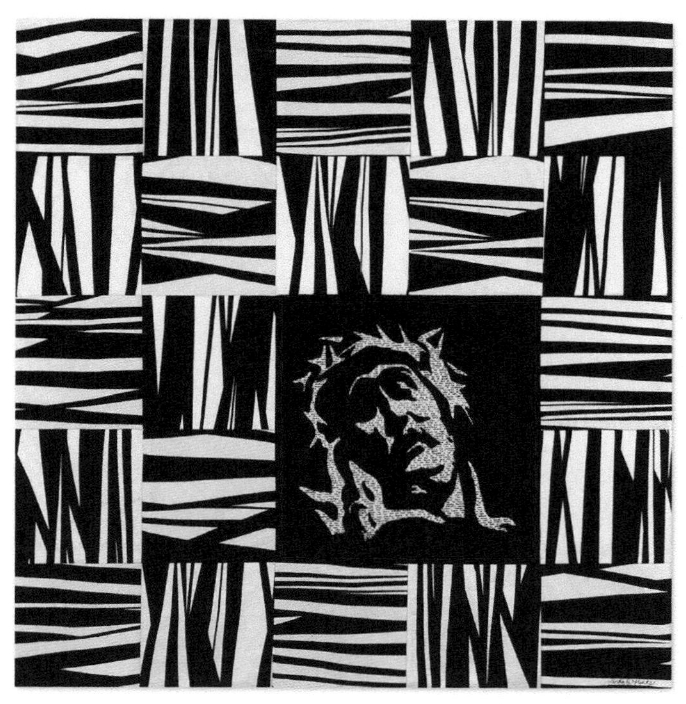

Linda W Henke
Indianapolis, IN, USA

Psalm 22 - Cross Road
37" x 37"

"My God, why have you forsaken me?" This work, inspired by the words of Psalm 22 that Jesus quoted from the cross, invites reflection on the cruciform quality of the call to Christian discipleship. When my own "cross road" is challenging, I too turn to the Psalms for comfort, courage, and strength.

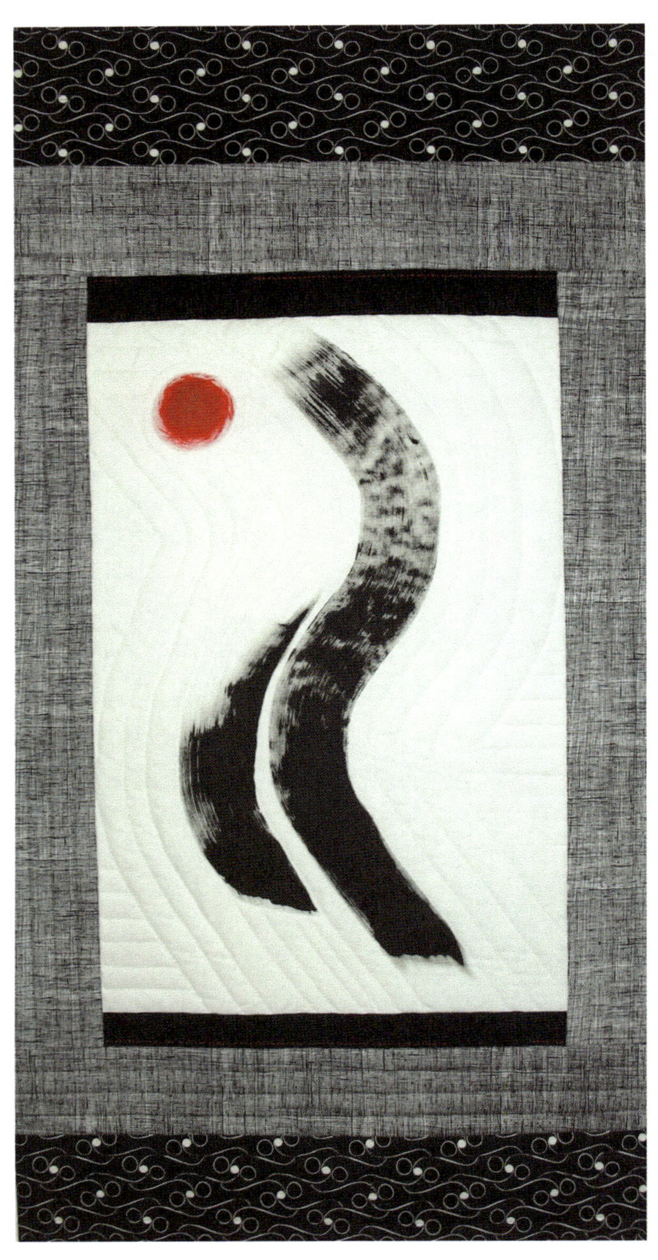

Linda A Miller
Culver City, CA, USA

Linear Moves
30" x 54"

I am inspired by the essential beauty in the ink calligraphy of Asian art traditions. Having worked with this meditative art form on paper, I wanted to translate the essence of the brushwork to cloth. By staying present with each step of painting and sewing, the process became a contemplative practice that allowed me to express the freshness of the moment in a direct way. To maintain simplicity in the overall presentation, I was influenced by the framing layouts of Asian scrolls in my arrangement of the borders.

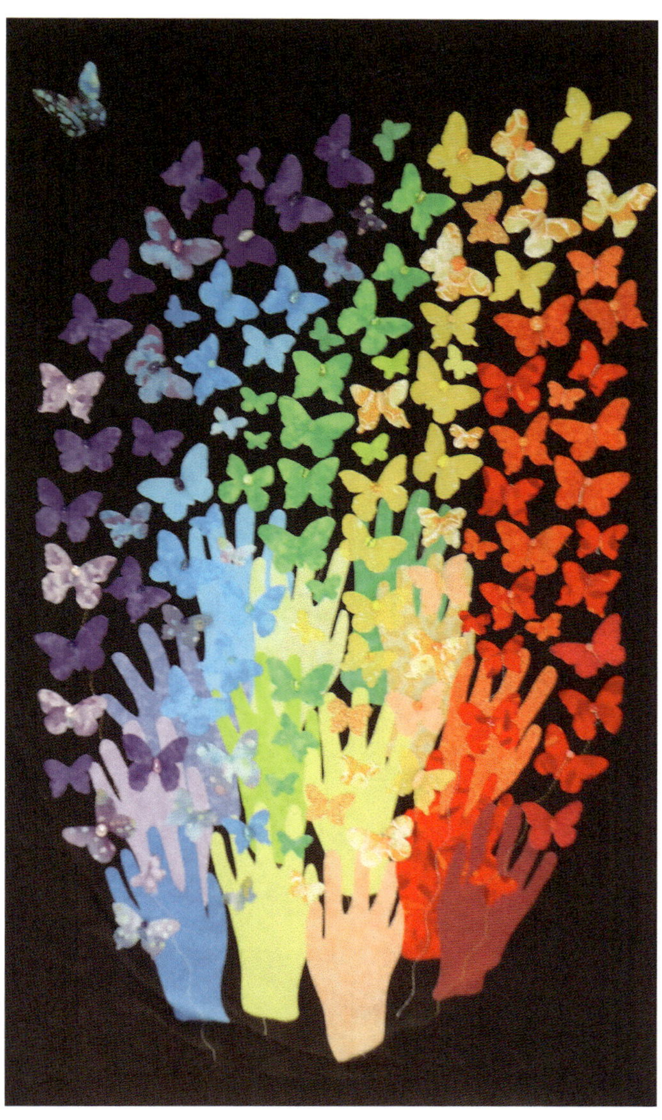

Linda K Bell
Supply, NC, USA

Life Is Change
22" x 34"

That is certainly true of my life which changed so dramatically in early 2008 with a diagnosis of Parkinson's Disease. And what is more emblematic of Change and Hope than a butterfly? Thus evolved this art quilt of a rainbow of butterflies,soaring up from open hands, symbolic of what I strive to create and my personal challenge, in the face of increasing physical limitations, to continue to do the handiwork that I so love. May this quilt lift your heart and spirit to soar upward on butterfly wings!

Salmos 90: 17
E seja sobre nós a
graca ao Senhor,
nosso Deus.
e confirma sobre
nos a obra das
nossas mãos.
sim, confirma a
obra das nossas
mãos.

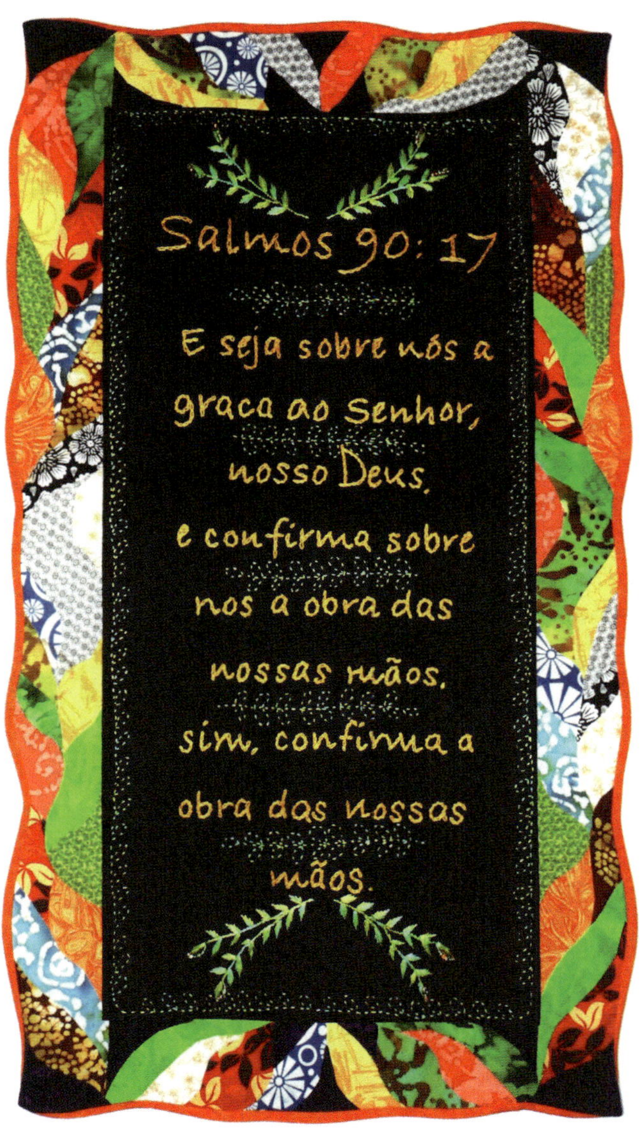

Beverly M Manuel
Indianapolis, IN, USA

Mozambique Memories
20" x 35"

I have just recently started quilting although I sewed as a young girl. I began quilting because I was going to Mozambique as part of a mission trip and thought it would be great to teach the ladies how to quilt while I was there. The quilt I taught them to make was a simple log cabin quilt and they did a great job. The border of this wall hanging is made from scraps left over from the quilt the ladies made. It will be sent to them as a gift.

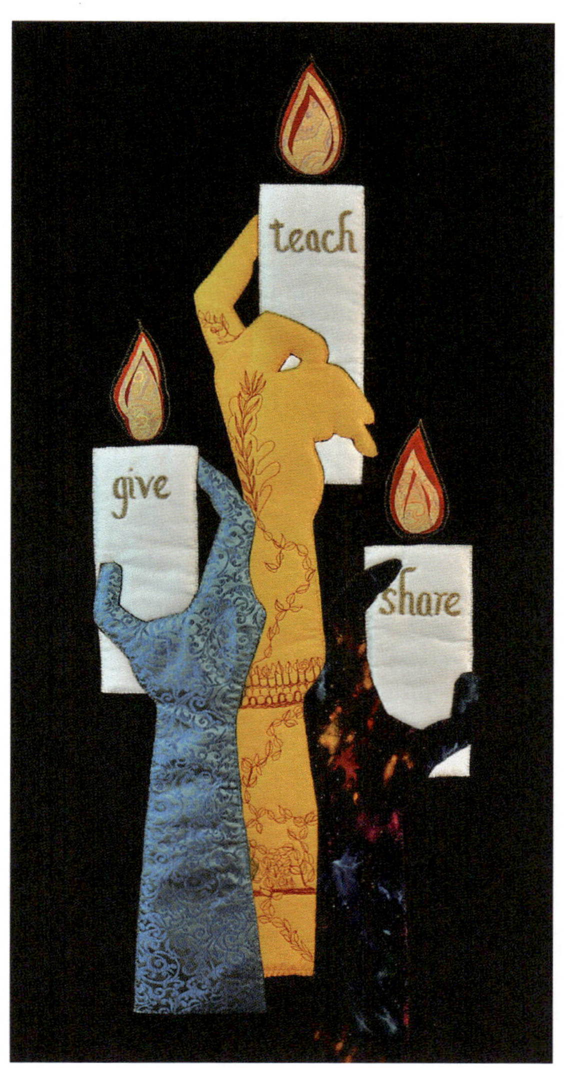

Suzanne Thompson
Ste Genevieve, MO, USA

Carry Your Candle #1: Give, Teach, Share
24" x 40"

This work is the first piece in a series inspired by a Chris Rice song. The chorus begins, "Carry your candle, go light your world." The words mean so much to me that I couldn't wait to share their essence through my art. With each new piece I strive to be the perfect party hostess. I offer simple, beautiful images to open a conversation that draws disparate people together in thoughtful discussion. I use these images, rather than narrative, because I find them more effective. Rather than presenting an explicit point of view, I just say, "Look!"

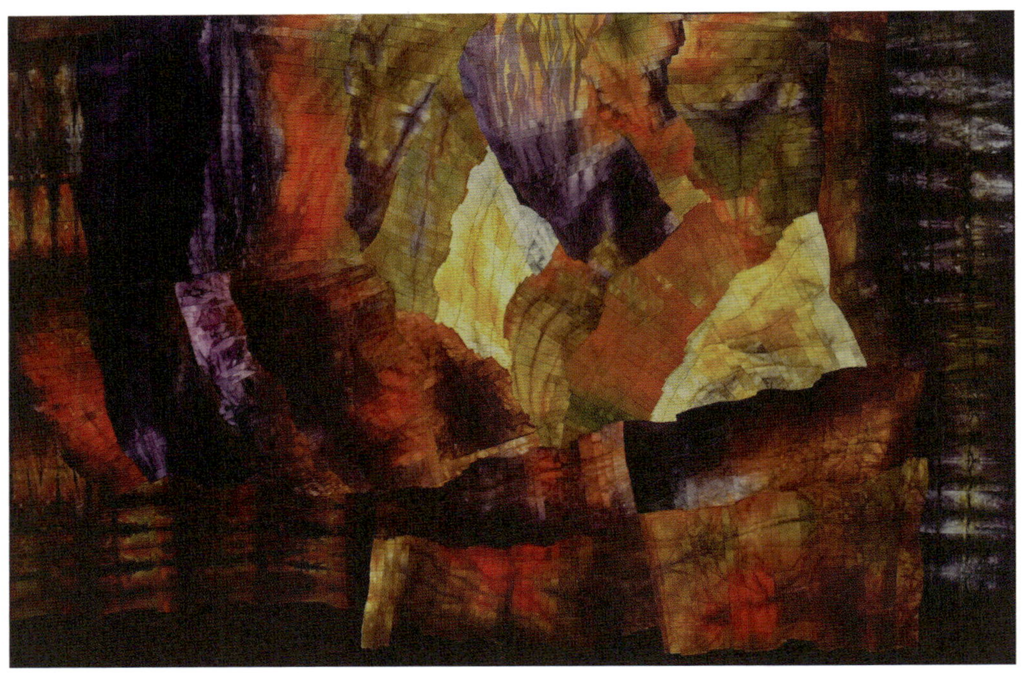

Donna Radner Chevy Chase, MD, USA
Twisting Canyons #7: On the Rim 59" x 38"

This quilt is part of a series inspired by the feelings evoked in me by the canyons and rock formations of the western United States. In this piece I was thinking of standing on the rim of the Grand Canyon and looking within in both a physical and spiritual sense. My reaction to the beauty and majesty of these vast natural structures and their eternal qualities is deeply spiritual. Their strength and endurance over time inspire me to emulate these qualities.

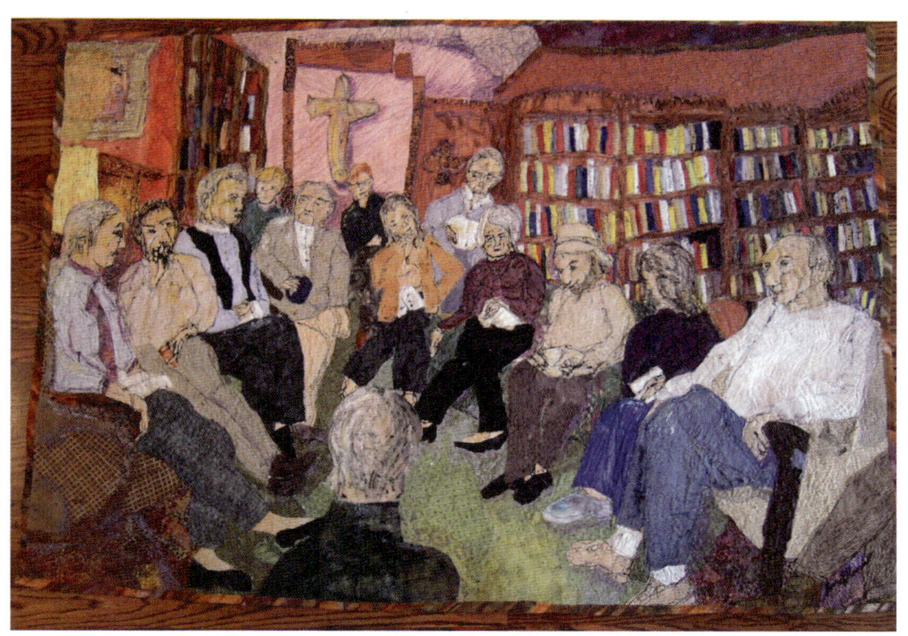

Jean Herman Denver, CO, USA
The Episcopalians 52" x 36"

Those of us that find inspiration through studying "the word" can identify with this serious group of searchers. I was part of a study group at my local church sketching each person as they learned and asked questions. The cross is paramount, but all the books are equally important. I learned to appreciate every person in the group, every question, every doubt, and yes every spark of inspiration that came from study and reflection. As we as humans look for God a group of like minded "searchers" can help us on our spiritual path.

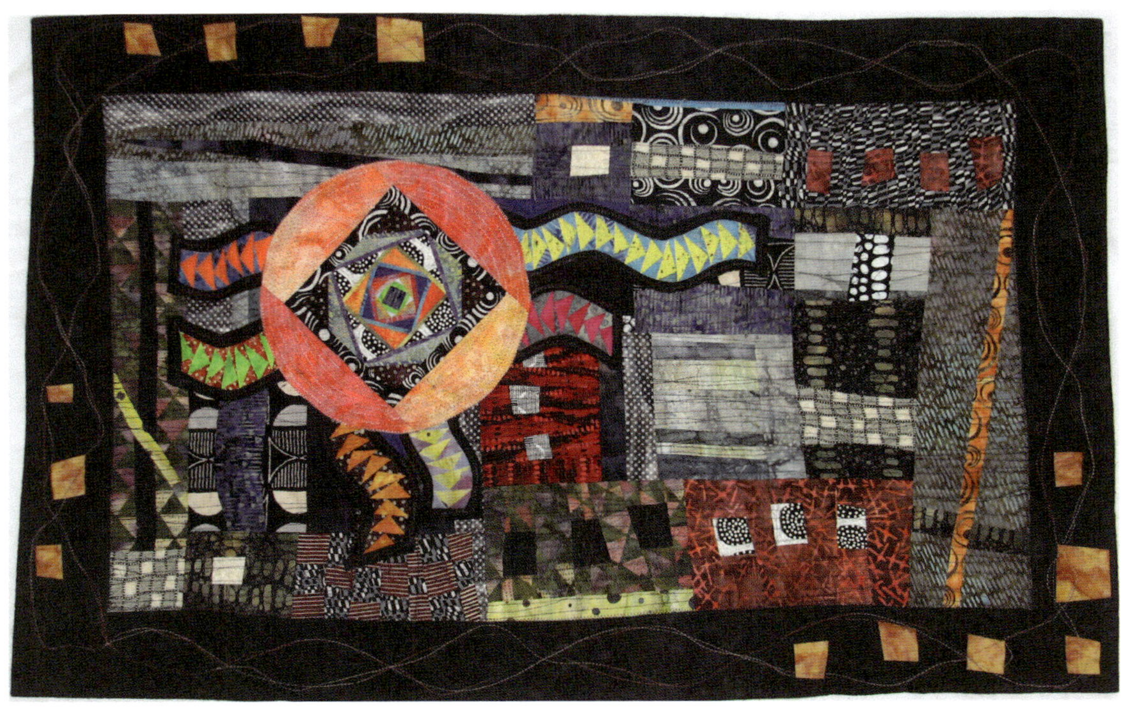

M. Camille Eaton Romig Barto, PA, USA
Zero/One–Reflecting on Universal Binary Language
34” x 21”

I was thinking and reading about proportional harmonies in the universe and the universal language of binary code. The Fibonacci numbers begin with 0 and 1 to create the golden rectangle’s harmonious spiral. Zero represents both nothingness and the totality in its empty circle form. One is considered to be a primordial unity, the beginning. Together, they create a primordial soup of dots and dashes, as seen in fabrics used in the quilt.

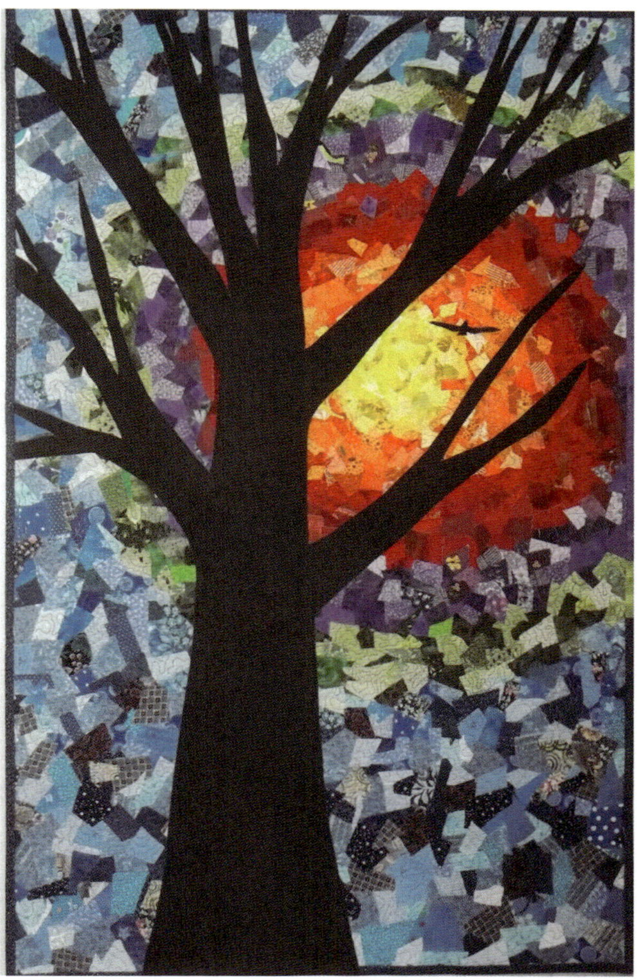

Eileen Kane
Oak Ridge, NC, USA

Soaring
23" x 34"

This piece is about taking a chance, facing a fear, making a choice, moving forward. We all have moments when we feel uncertain, unsure or even fearful. But it takes courage to take that first step, make that first flight, take that next chance, make that decision. Once that step is taken, may you soar - soar through your troubles or fears or obstacles. See where the wind takes you.

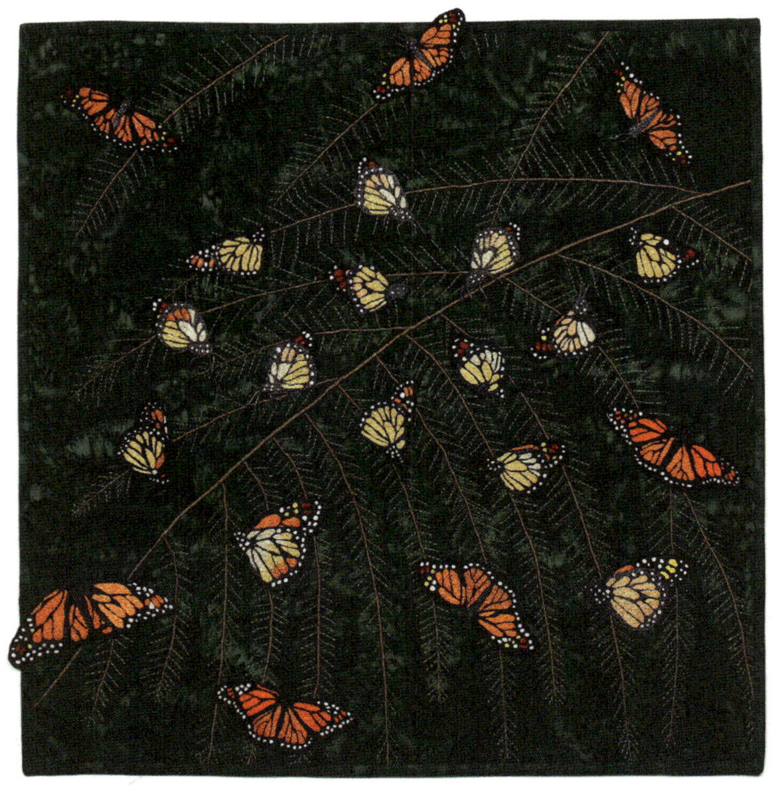

Naomi Weidner
Albany, OR, USA

Monarch Butterflies
20" x 20"

Monarch butterflies (Danaus plexippus) are an inspiration to me. How can something that weighs less than a paperclip leave its summer home in eastern Canada or U.S., and fly over 1500 miles to somewhere it has never been - the wintering grounds in the highlands of central Mexico? Once on their wintering grounds, the Monarchs cluster together to stay warm on oyamel fir trees (Abies religiosa). In mid-March the same Monarchs end their hibernation and begin migrating north. They lay eggs before they die, leaving to future generations the rest of the northward migration and all of the return migration.

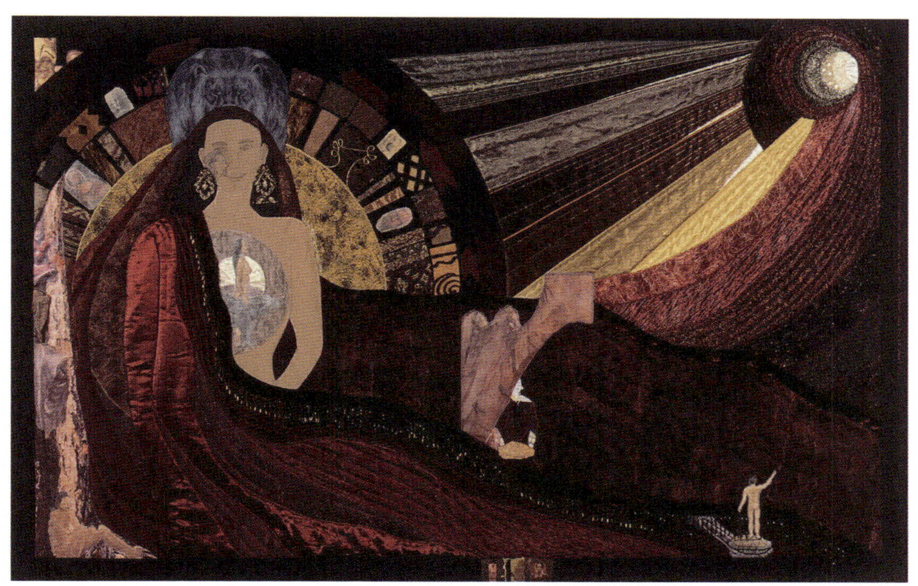

Linda K Filby-Fisher Overland Park, KS, USA
Dignity: Celebration of Life Series 69.5" x 44"

The power of the earth surges up
Through the soles of your feet.
Ancient rhythms resonate in your blood
Calling your name.
You stand as the tree stands,
Your feet grounded by stones,
Your back lifted with promise!
Created with thanksgiving for
The life force of all beings—of
All generations!

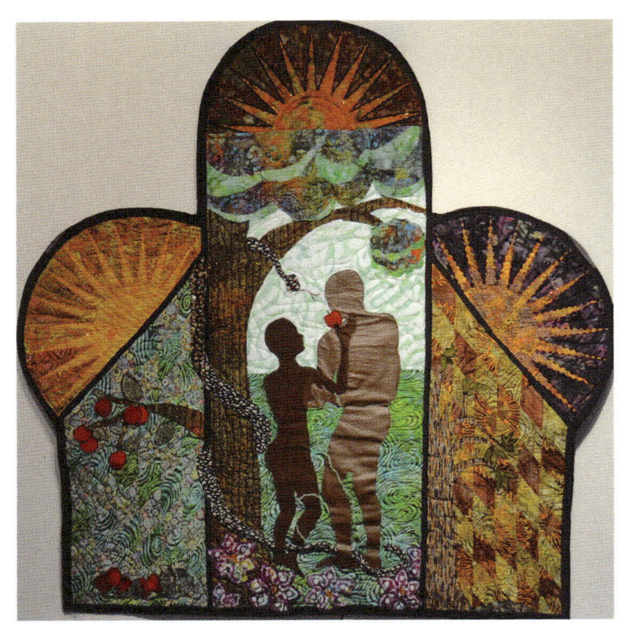

Lydia Allen-Berry
Philadelphia, PA, USA

Adam & Eve
40" x 40"

I have always been fascinated with Adam and Eve, imagining how perfect life would be had they remained in the utopia of the Garden of Eden, and wondering at what power could tempt them to defiance. This triptych, fashioned in the style of a stained glass window, depicts Adam & Eve on the brink, where all the potency, promise, and seduction of the choice begin to be comprehended. The consequences await...

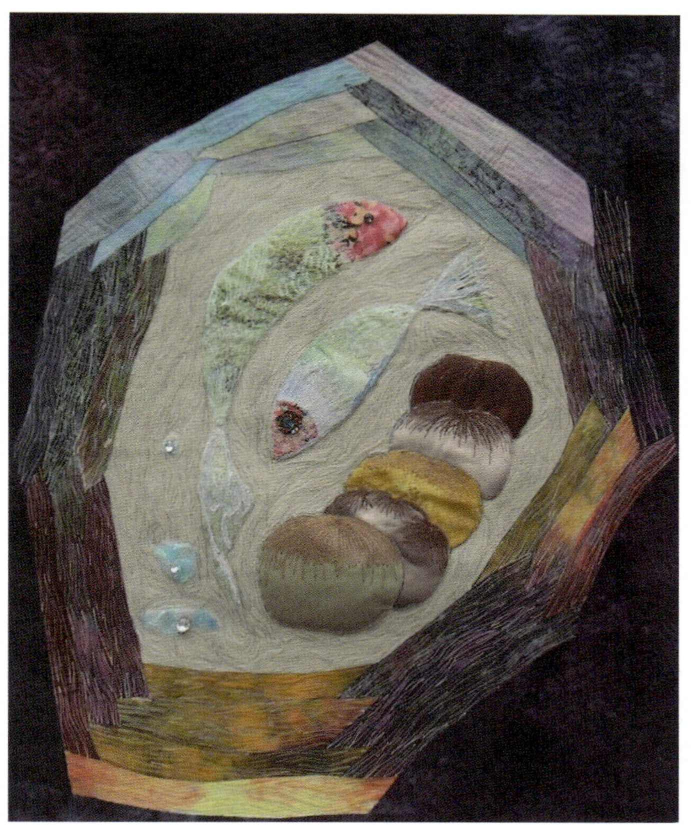

Annabel R Barber
Tealby, Lincs

Sustenance
22.5” x 26”

This quilt shows the loaves and fishes from the feeding of the 5000, one of the greatest miracles. Christ takes the simple food a child offers, blesses it and feeds those who are hungry. We each have our gifts, our loaves and fishes that can feed the world, both physically and spiritually. But it takes courage to offer something of ourselves, to come to Jesus and give him what we have and allow him to use it for others. And too often our society seems to be saying "But I want a burger and fries, not loaves and fish!"

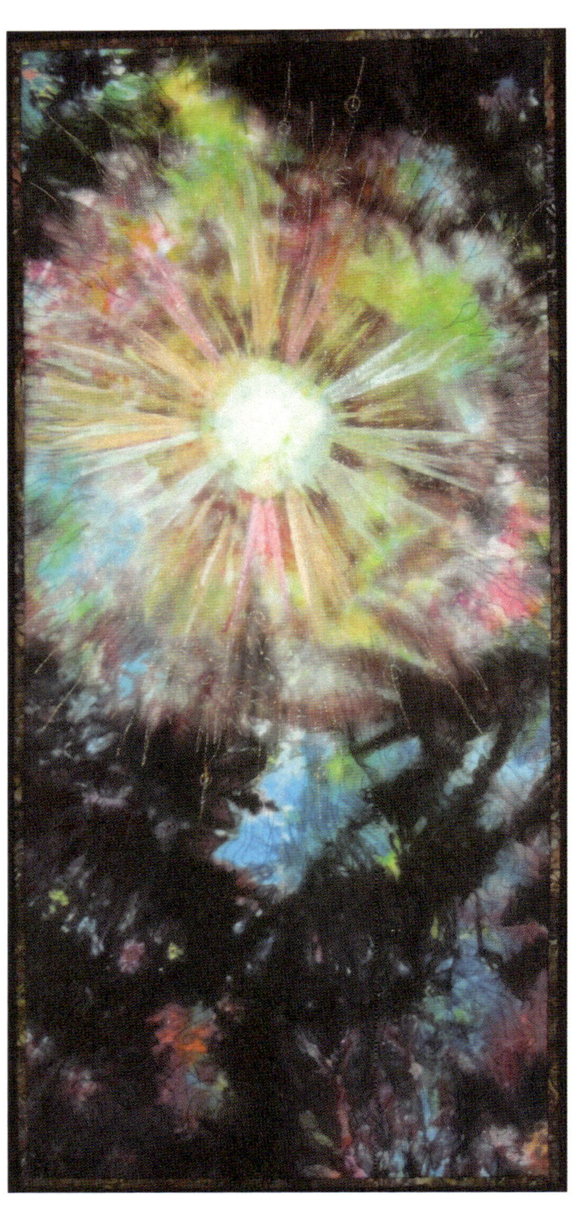

Ginnie Hebert
Puyallup, WA, USA

Light of the World II
17.5" x 37"

Aging/Dying/Living On
"We are a way for the universe to know itself. Some part of our being knows this is where we came from. We long to return. And we can, because the cosmos is also within us. We're made of star stuff." Carl Sagan

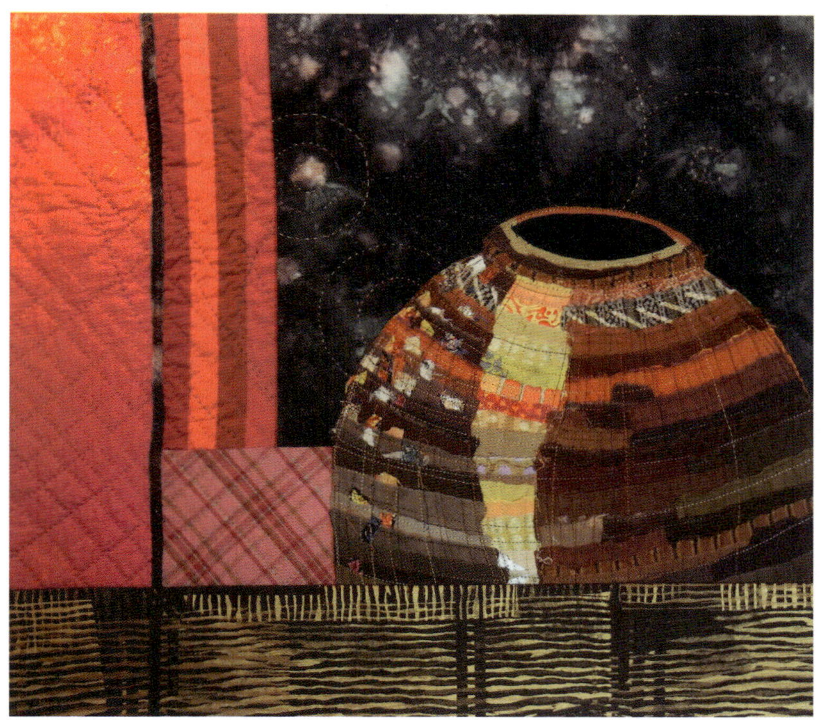

Eleanor Levie Philadelphia, PA, USA
Vessel 23" x 20"

My mother was the vessel for my existence, and she remains the source for my sense of how to live and love. She is inspired to work in clay--and lets fire and serendipity take over. I am inspired to work in fabric and thread--and increasingly let the piece tell me where it should go. For both of us, the greatest satisfaction and success come from quick playful dashes rather than planned determination and over-labored technique. So perhaps the surprise and mystery of the process is the greatest source of the C/creator's divine spark.

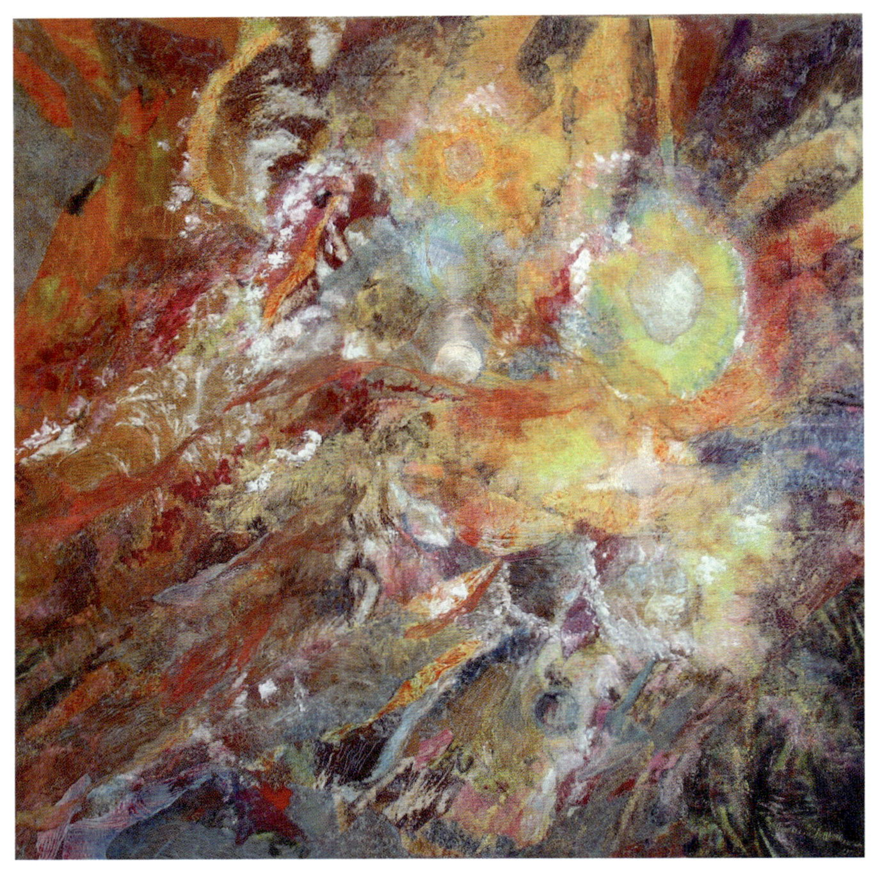

Marianne R Williamson Miami, FL, USA
Big Bang 52" x 51"

The concept of an event as monumental as the "Big Bang" is so far from my understanding, but it has inspired me to make a number of pieces about the cosmos.

PEACE/ BROTHERHOOD

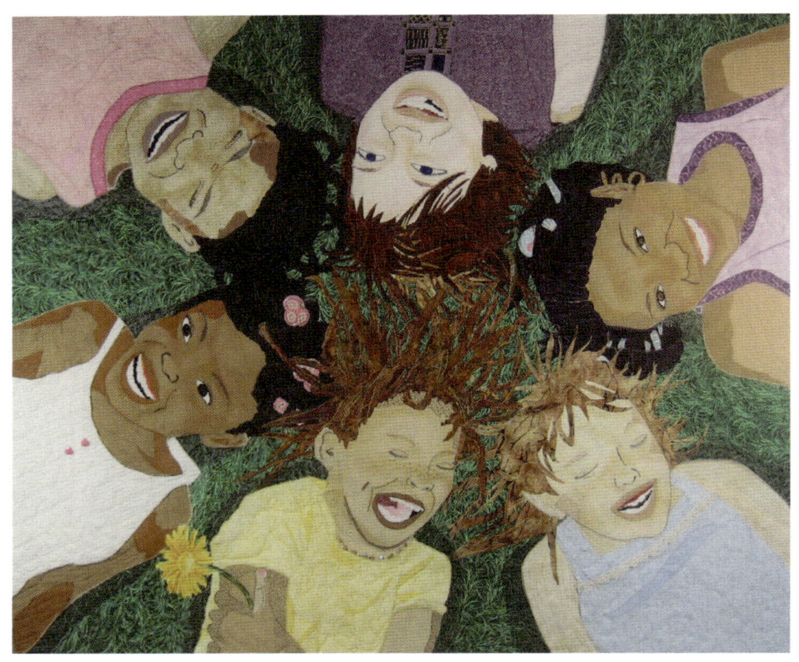

Susan Walen Bethesda, MD, USA
FRIENDS: May Our Children Do Better Than We Did 37" x 30.5"

In 2006 I found a photo of 6 little girls lying in the grass, giggling. I was captivated by the photo and got permission from the photographer, James Levine, to use it. At that point, my skills weren't up to the task.

In 2010, I was invited to make a quilt for a show on Racism, and shortly stumbled on that old newspaper photo. It made me grin and I thought that if we could overcome racism, this is what it would look like.

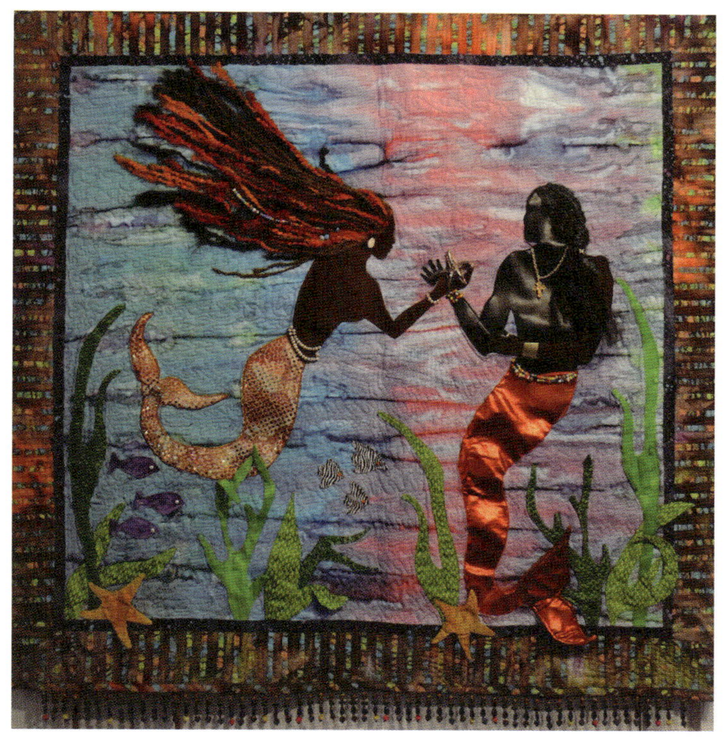

Lydia Allen-Berry
Philadelphia, PA, USA

Yemaya Calming Olokun
36" x 36"

In the Yoruba pantheon of deities there is Yemaya, mother of the sea, and Olokun, the storm-maker, god of the lower depths of the ocean. Often appearing in the form of a mermaid and merman, Yemaya is a creative force and protector of man while Olokun is a destructive force who unleashes violent storms and powerful hurricanes to punish man. When reflecting on Yemaya and Olokun, I am intrigued that Yemaya alone has the power to calm Olokun. This quilt depicts the interplay between turbulence and calm, male and female energy, and the vengeful and loving nature of God. Being of Yoruba descent,it also represents the common threads in my religious heritage.

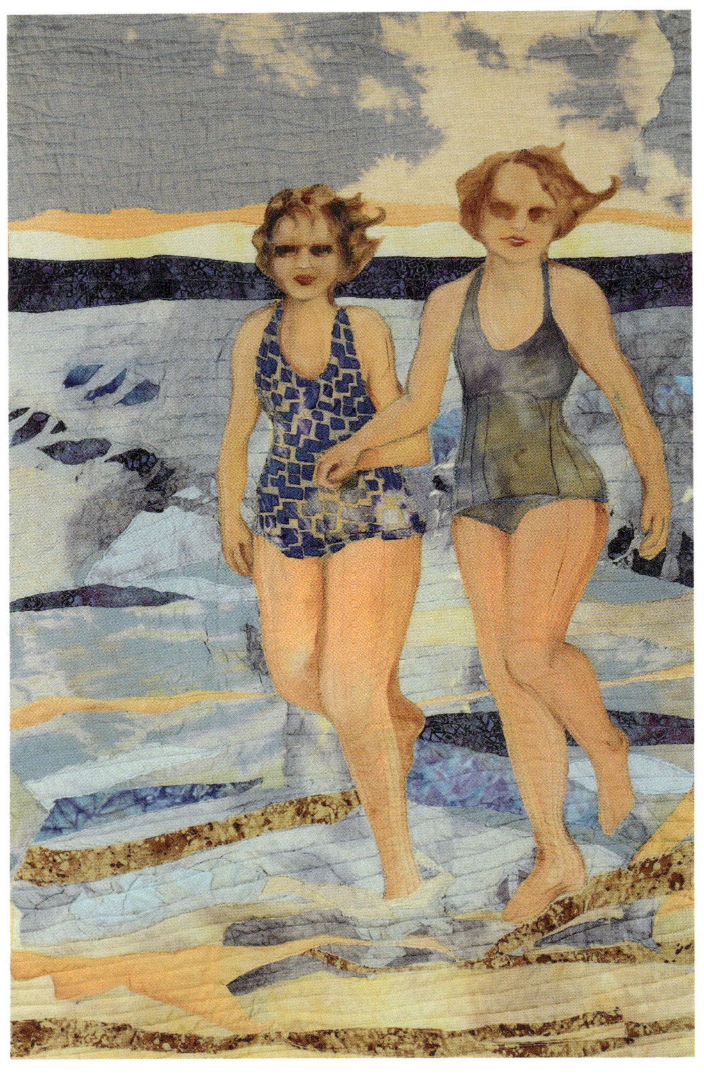

Sharon Tesser
Lawrenceburg, IN, USA

A Day At The Beach
32" x 39"

There is nothing more beautiful or powerful in my life than sisterhood. The peace that comes from knowing there is someone to walk through this life with makes every incident manageable. Peace comes from the support and love shared between people who would do anything, be anything , give anything, to make the path easier. This life journey is a gift that is better shared.

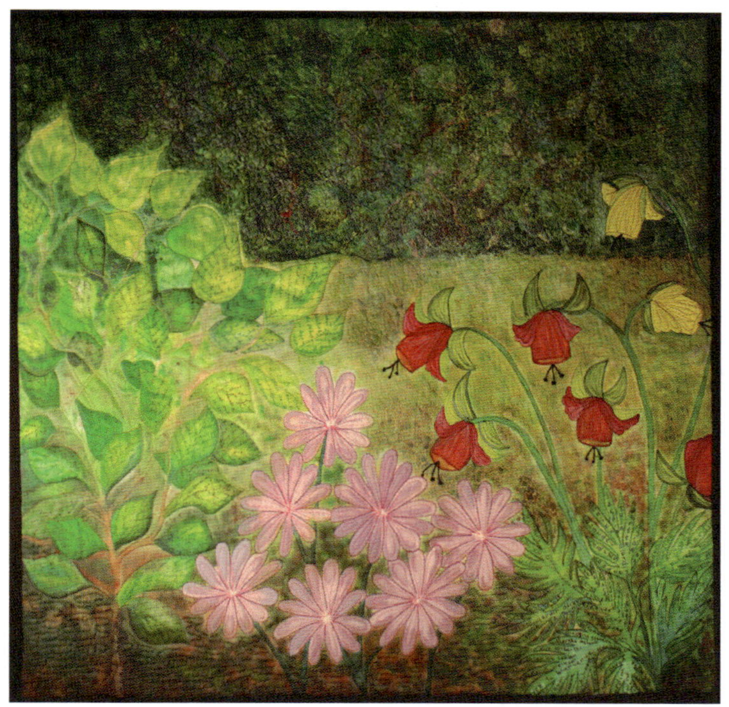

Barb Forrister
Austin, TX, USA

Welcome to My Garden
34” x 33”

Welcome to My Garden beckons visitors to enter and gather inspirational phrases as if they were flowers. The leaves on the right bear the words, "welcome" and "garden" in languages including French, German, Italian, Swahili, Spanish, and Norwegian.. Phrases on the leaves of the plants to the left include messages about special time with friends and family, secrets whispered, conversations and intimate moments from long ago. The tranquilt scene evokes a time I walked through the garden, hand in hand with my lover or shared a cup of tea with my best friend. I remember back to my own childhood memories and the sensations when I first walked through grass and felt the blades between my toes or breathed the scent of a favorite flower. It is here I am reminded of the past, and where I have learned to dream.

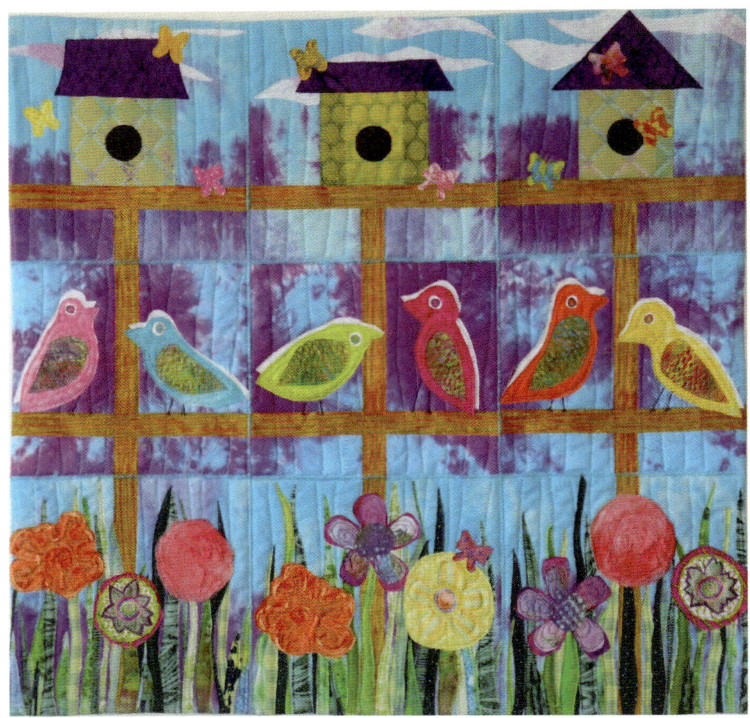

Brenda Schlechter
Largo, Fl, USA

Friends in the Garden
29" x 29"

Friends in the Garden portrays an idyllic scene of peace and brotherhood among friends. This neighborhood with its well tended gardens and houses is home to birds of different colors, and perhaps a variety of cultural backgrounds. Despite their differences the birds are happily getting along with each other, something we could all learn. By using brilliant color, simple shapes, and a basic organic scene. I hope to convey my optimism that this scene can be a learning tool for all. That we can all learn to get along.

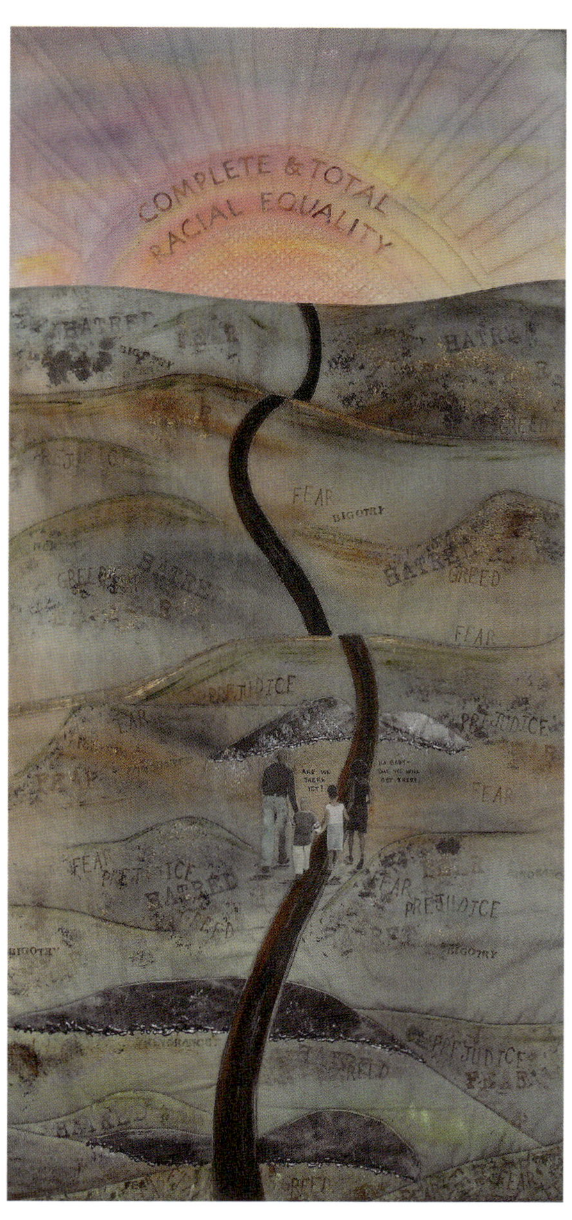

Sherry Boram
Pendleton, IN, USA

Journey
22" x 44"

The election of the first African American President, Barack Obama, seems to have revived issues about race relations in our country. Using journey as a metaphor, a young family travels the long and difficult road to equality as United States citizens of color. I hope thought and dialog result from those who view my art.

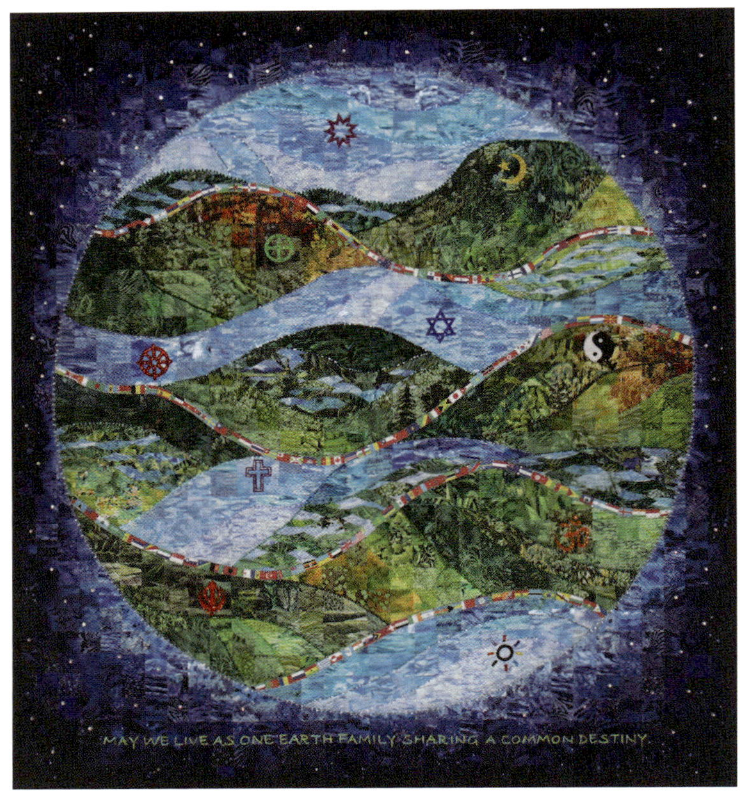

Lin Schiffner
Nevada City, CA, USA

Earth Prayer
32" x 33.5"

My sacred journey, including my art, is dedicated to fostering peace, compassion, and mutual understanding among people sharing this planet. The piece expresses my prayer for Earth - the vast, beautiful and abundant home that we share with a diversity of life and cultures, represented by the flags of the world nations and symbols of major religions. Humanity living in peace and harmony, appreciating and embracing our differences with compassion and respect, will allow our planet to thrive. The central theme is "May we live as one earth family sharing a common destiny" which is hand-embroidered on the piece.

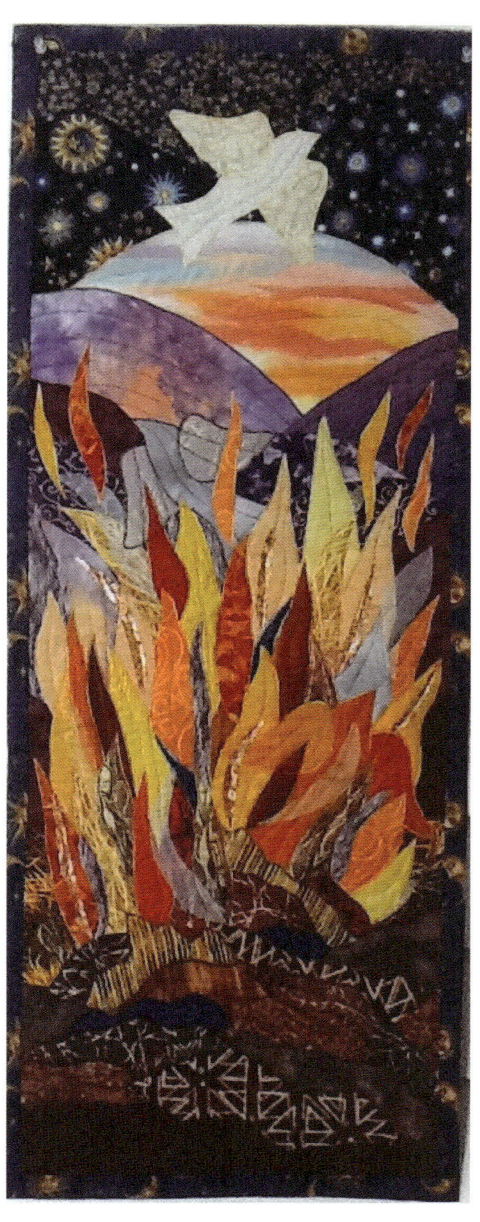

Kit J Tossmann
Louisville, KY, USA

Peace Rising
17” x 40”

I started this piece some time ago and got stuck. Unable to get it to work the way I envisioned, I almost felt like actually burning it. Instead I quit, rolled it up, and put it away. While reorganizing my studio space I rediscovered it and decided to re-visit the piece. I found that I had learned so much more, that I was able to resurrect it! The inspiration for it came out of feeling that even in the midst of chaos, strife and turmoil, peace is in there somewhere striving to emerge. We battle internal and external wars of all kinds and are bombarded by threats around us every day. Around the world there are still too many people fighting. My hope is that somehow, someday peace will arise and prevail.

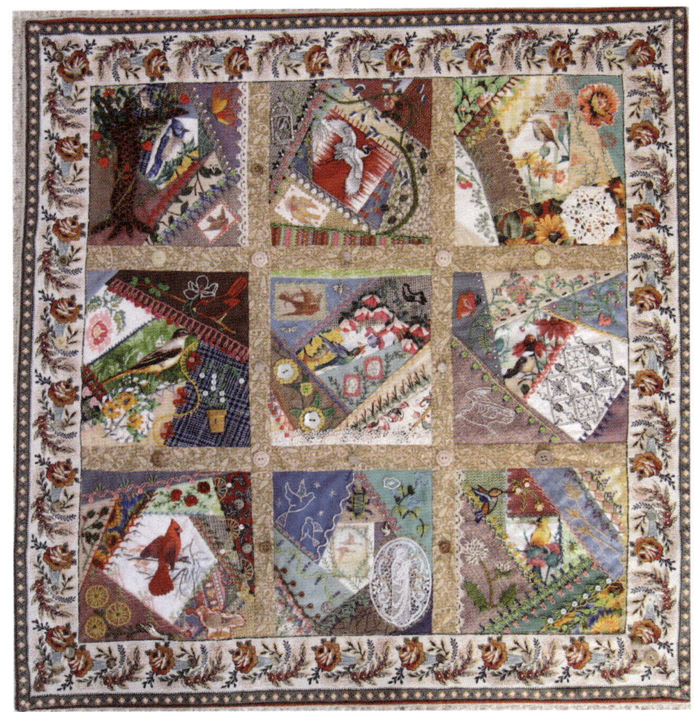

Barbara B Curiel
Arcata, CA, USA

Saint Francis Preaches to the Birds
32" x 33"

Saint Francis of Assisi was the son of a rich family who rejected all worldly goods and recognized the brotherhood not only between people of different social ranks, but between people and animals as well. There are many stories of Francis speaking to animals and of them responding to him. In one frequently told story, he preaches to the birds, and they are his attentive and responsive listeners. I like to think that these stories demonstrate the dignity of all beings and I decided to render it in a crazy quilt, an embellished form that frequently features birds.

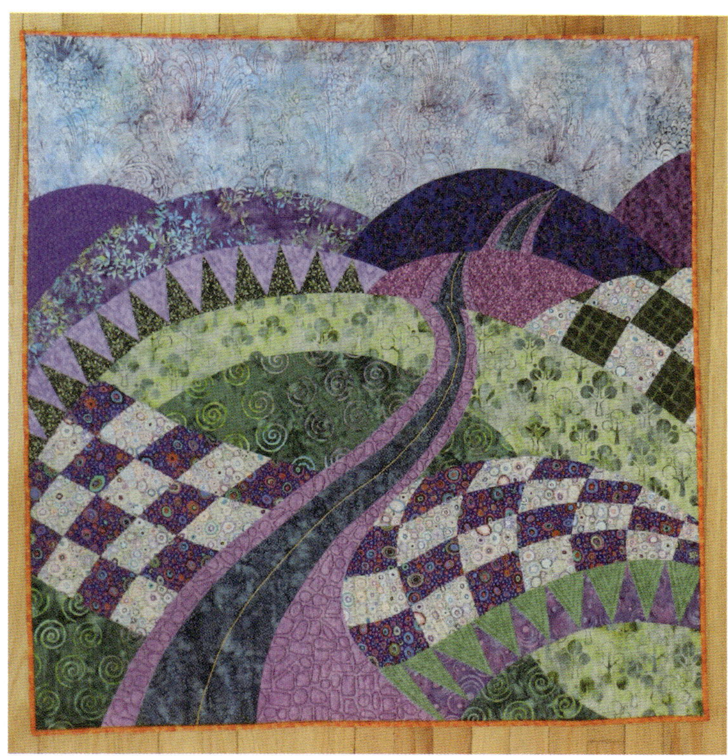

Maggie Ward
Warrenton, VA, USA

Route 211
39.5” x 40”

Far away from the DC suburbs, away from the crowds and the stress, Route 211 winds its quiet way toward the Blue Ridge. This is where I go when I need to think, to feel comforted, to leave behind failure or frustration or loss. The hills rise and fall in their own rhythm. One can see civilization's thumbprint in the tidy fields and ordered vineyards, but out here nature and humanity co-exist in peace. I ride through the landscape and I am renewed.

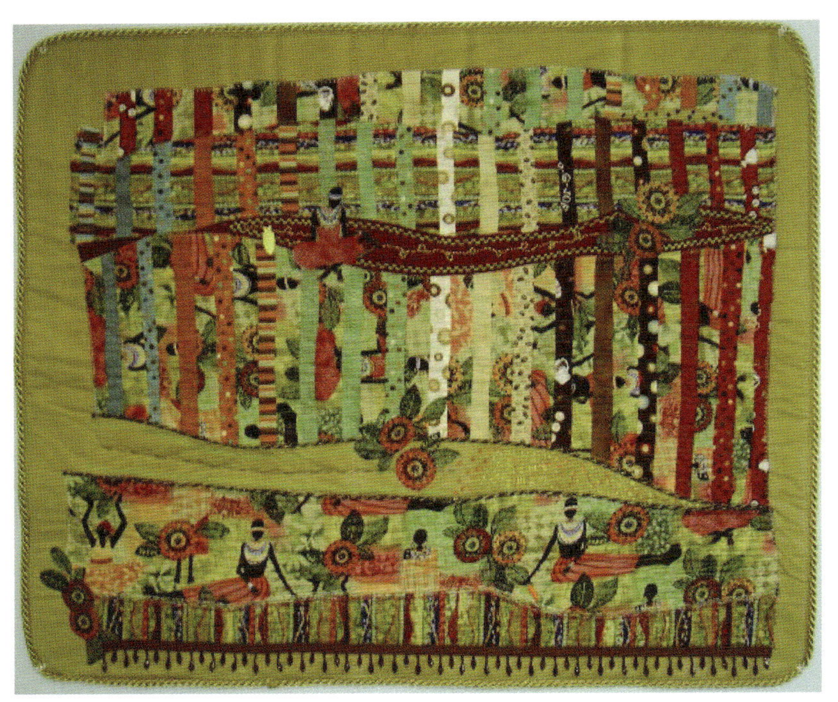

Sharon H Bailey Cabot, AR, USA
Freedom Within the Boundaries 39.50” x 36.50”

In creating “Freedom Within the Boundaries”, I reflected on my missionary friends' experience with the Masai women in East Kenya in the 1970s. Since the advent of Christian missionaries, there is no longer fear of perversion to these women from their tribal Witch Doctors. Fabrics and embellishments and layering are my favorite expressions of creativity as well as part of my sacred journey.

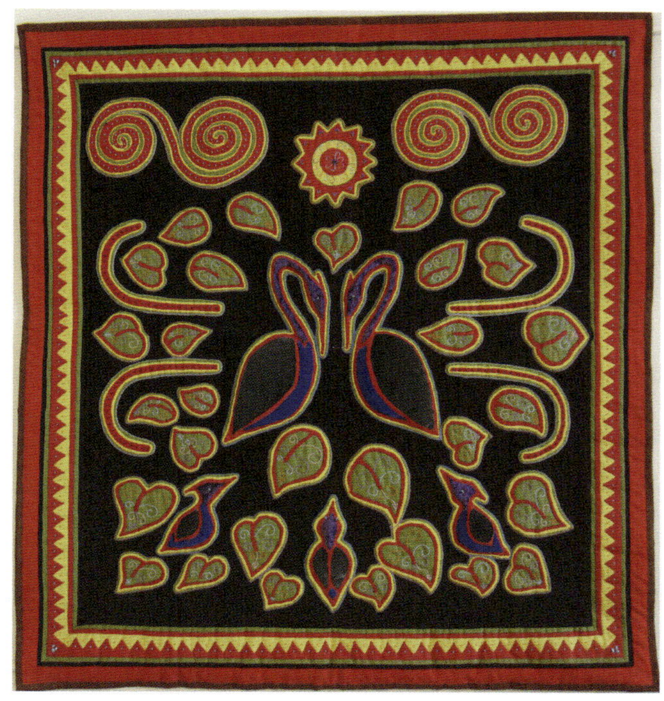

Hélène Blanchet
Calgary, Alberta, Canada

La Famille
38"" x 42""

This piece represents faith in family. The herons sit high in a tree in the safety of their home. The tree reaches its branches around them in a loving embrace. The parents sit protectively over the chicks who look to them for guidance. The tree is the Tree of Life that supports them. The sun allows all life to exist. The cloud spirals represent ancestors and generations to come. The multi-layered borders provide barriers to keep negative elements away from the safety of their home. The herons are adorned in velvet to represent the richness of the soul and in colours that reflect their strength. Blue is the purity of the heart with which they were born. Green is the integrity and the natural world that keeps us grounded. Purple is the wisdom that life will impart on them. Red is for the passion that makes us feel truly alive. Yellow is the day and represents energy and activity. Black is the night and represents contemplation and quiet.

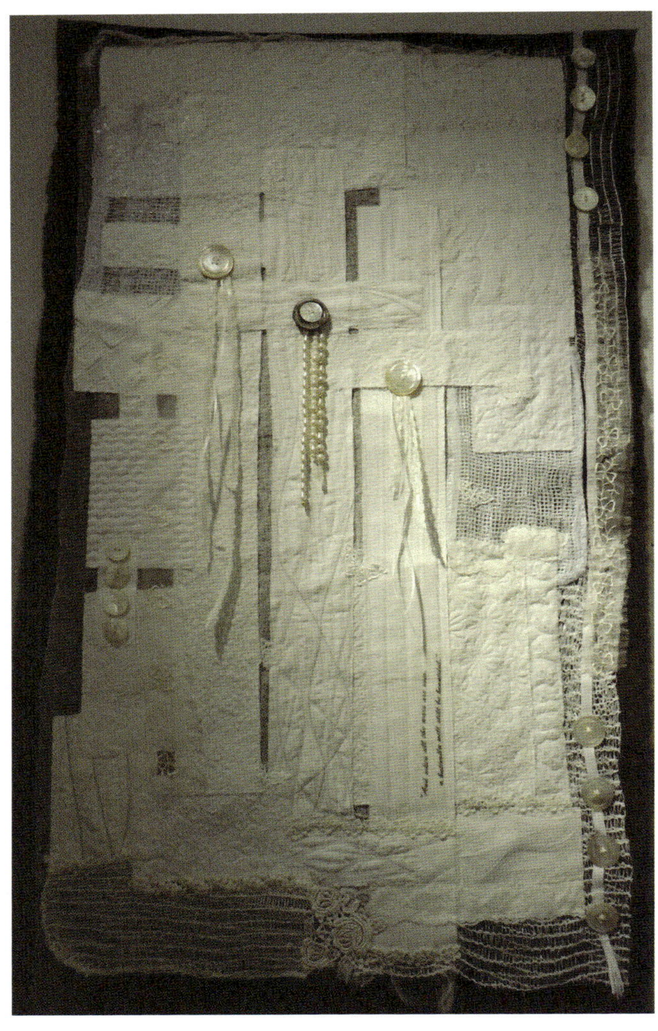

Barbara K Boatman
Alexandria, VA, USA

Butterflies for Peace
24” x 39”

My artistic goal is to use recycled materials in unexpected ways. This piece was created to convey the wastefulness of war. The natural world is peaceful. War is unnatural, a loud event created by man. No matter the reason for any war, when it's over the world eventually goes back to a peaceful state. All we gain are lost souls. In this piece I see a cemetery of crosses shrouded by clouds of early morning fog. I see a fragile world holding itself together against the dark. "And when all the wars are over, a butterfly will still be beautiful".

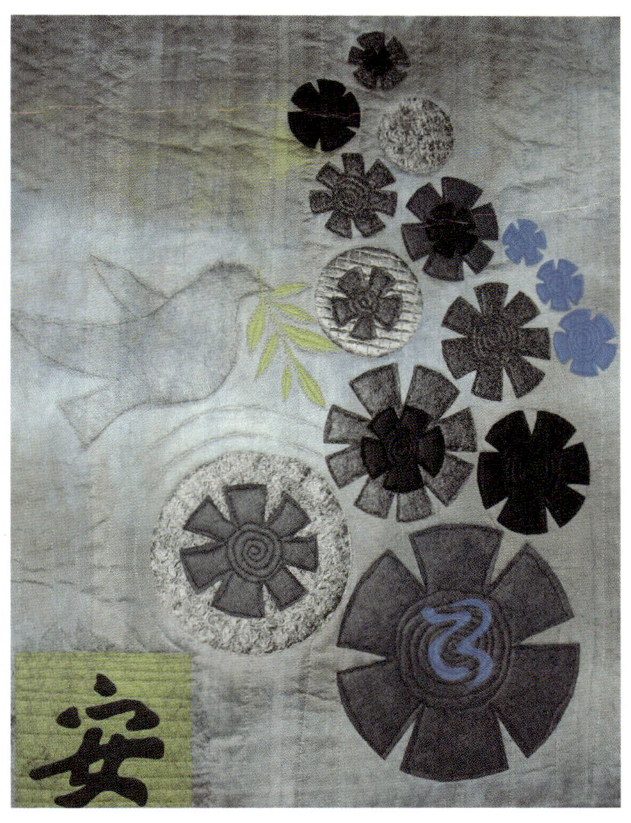

Amalia P Morusiewicz
Mitchellville, MD, USA

Peaceful Passage
24” x 32”

How often can we thank a towing company for inspiring art? The chaos of my life increased when my car was towed. The peaceful dove with olive branch represents the friend and her young son who offered me a ride. The Chinese character for peace, is shadowed, as there was calm in the chaos. Through this simple gesture of a ride, I was granted peaceful passage that day. I remind myself to help make this passage through life more peaceful for others and myself. Chaos surrounds us always and having that inner peace will allow us safe passage.

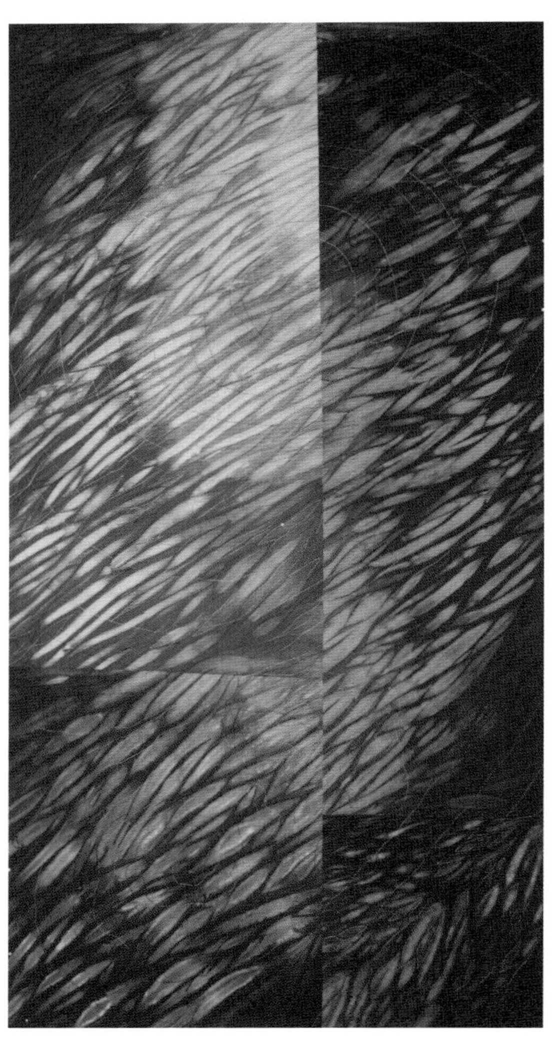

Catherine L Waltz
Fort Lauderdale, FL, USA

Water (Vortex Series)
26" x 49"

Peace. I descend with scuba tanks on my back, a mask and regulator in my mouth. I exit a short tunnel and hang seemingly in mid-air, suspended alongside a cliff. For a moment I am breathless and all is incredibly quiet. Water below me becomes darker. Light from above me slices through the blue water. The light is broken by the movement of the surge and my motions making its own paths of wiggling light. All is peaceful as I drift along the face of The Wall. (West Bay, Cayman Islands, 1986).

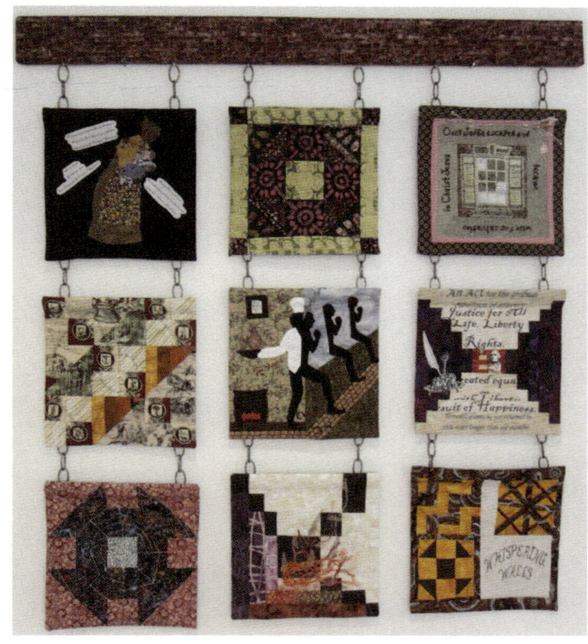

SherriJoyce King
Gladwyne, PA, USA

Whispering Walls
40” x 48”

The truth is stark, the irony undeniable - the first President of a new democracy founded on principles of freedom and equality, was a slaveholder. George Washington kept nine people enslaved as domestic servants in our first White House, in Philadelphia: Oney Judge, Moll, Austin, Hercules, Richmond, Giles, Paris, Christopher Sheels, and Joe Richardson. Quarterly Quilters, a group of Philadelphia quilt artists, collaborated to present "Whispering Walls," nine independently quilted blocks suspended by chains, each block honoring an enslaved inhabitant of the President's House. With fabric and thread, we celebrate the humanity, individual dignity, and courageous brotherhood of these nine slaves. Quarterly Quilters also include Michelle Flamer, Susan Levering, Sally Poulshock, Linda Rosenstein, Jo Countley, Corrie Roberts, Susan Sandler.

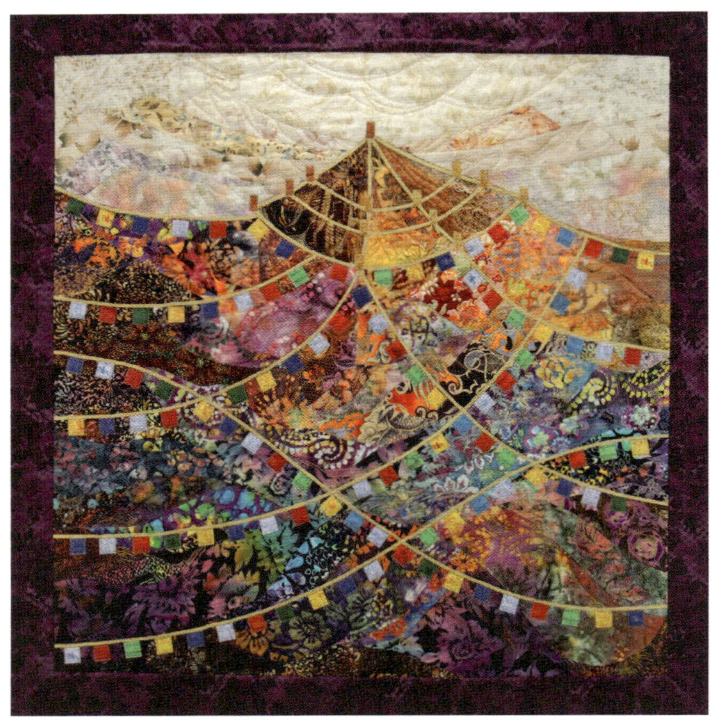

Peg Green
Reston, VA, USA

Tibetan Prayer Flags
43" x 43"

In Tibetan Buddhist tradition, prayer flags are hung outdoors in the open air to send out prayers for peace, love, and compassion to bless the whole world. As the flags, which contain prayers written in Sanskrit, are blown by the wind, their prayers sanctify the air and spread good will across all pervading space. I am inspired by this way of being prayerful, and I love the beauty of the colorful flags.

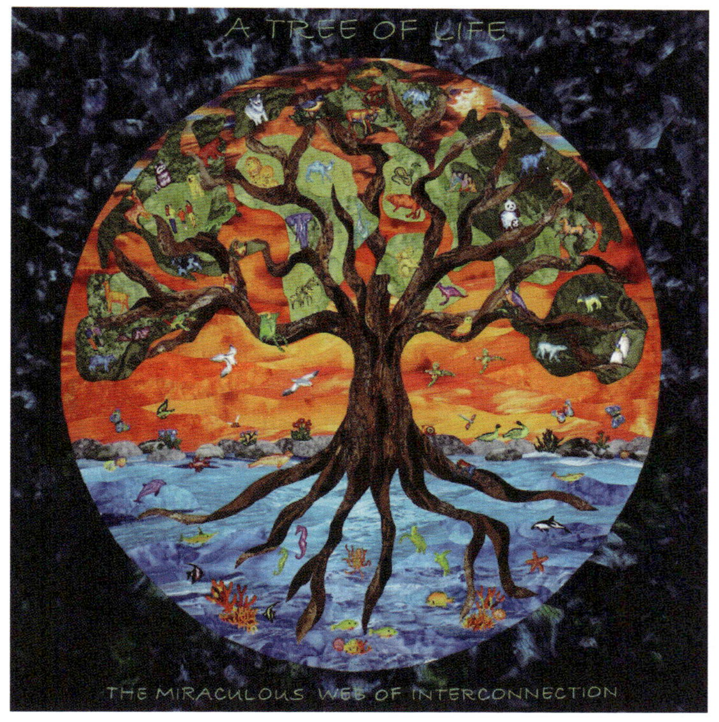

Lin Schiffner
Nevada City, CA, USA

A Tree of Life
32" x 32"

My art is a reflection of a sacred journey that includes exploring concepts of life that unites humanity and embraces the sanctity of our existence on Earth. This piece honors the miracle of life – the web of interconnection among life forms and elements on Earth. The continents are represented as foliage and the creatures are loosely linked to where they may live. Although only a tiny leaf on the tree, human beings are responsible for its future. May we learn to protect, cherish, nourish and preserve the Tree of Life so it may grow in peace, harmony and love.

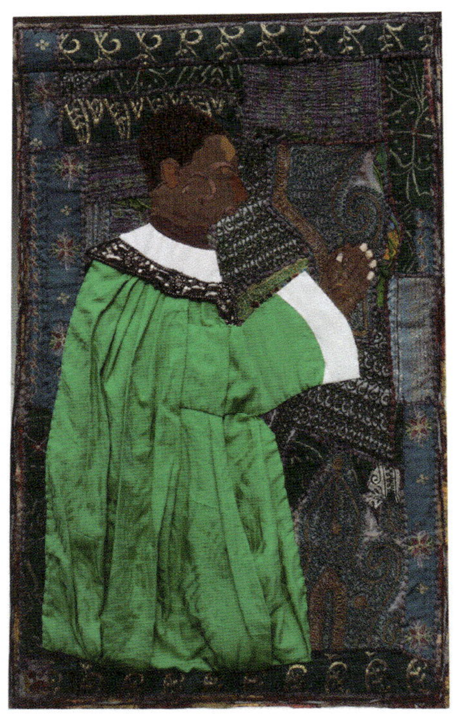

Sonia M Callahan
Piedmont, CA, USA

Universality of Prayer
21.5" x 34.5"

In most of the major religions of the world there are threads of commonality which involve prayer, offering and reflection.. It is my hope that the these common traits can bring us together rather than separate us in a world where peace and brotherhood are badly needed. While we chose our form of worship, we can also choose to recognize forms of worship to which others are equally dedicated. Through greater understanding of the diversity of religions our world can become more peaceful.The fabrics used in this quilt originate in Africa, India, Europe and the Americas and they join together to create a universal image. Perhaps this quilt will stimulate thought on religious tolerance.

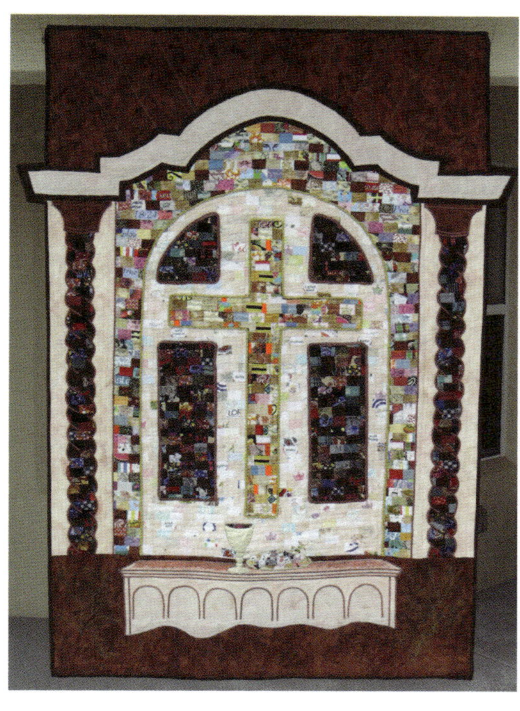

Susan C Clayton
Port Orange, FL, USA

Sanctuary Quilt
50" x 67"

Our congregation received a grant from the Lilly Foundation, part of which was to be used for a sanctuary banner. We have a Spanish mission style church, and we chose to replicate the carved cross in the chancel. The congregation contributed fabric that had personal meaning, and we received fabrics such as traffic vests, baby bibs, letter jackets, military symbols, a wedding dress, and lots of t-shirts. For our congregation, this quilt has become a symbol of who we are. We are the Body of Christ, as represented by the seemingly incongruent fabrics, tied together by the love of God

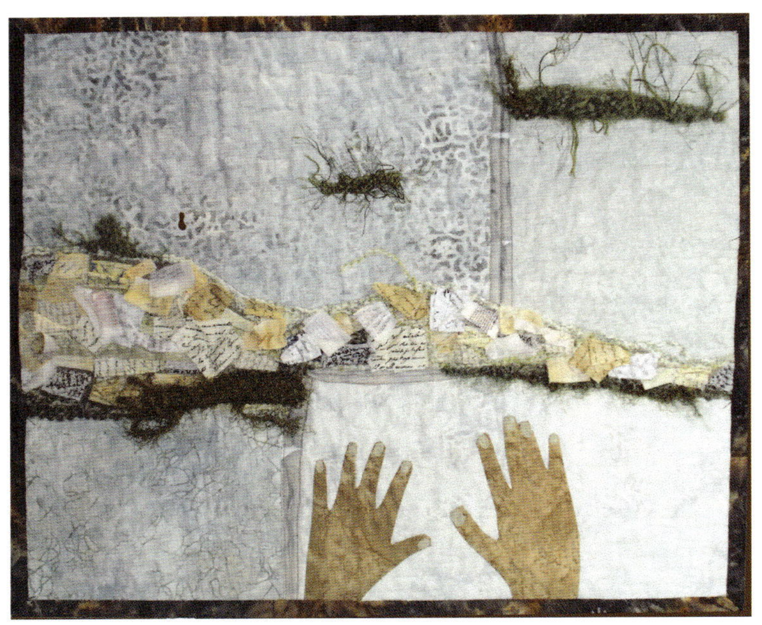

Barbara J Mitchell Birmingham, AL, USA
Prayers at the Wailing Wall 31" x 25"

On a recent trip to Israel, I spent time at the Wailing Wall in Jerusalem. This has been a place of pilgrimage for centuries, and many people leave written prayer notes tucked into cracks between stones. I witnessed people of various nationalities and languages praying at this location; prayers were silent, verbal, or physical with hands placed against the wall. It was a privilege and honor to share a time of prayer with others; I imagined prayers being offered for families, health, safety, and peace. I was reminded how our prayers unite us wherever and whoever we are.

Beloved community
May all beings be well
LOVE
Seek justice, love mercy
Blessed are the poor
Blessed are those who are generous

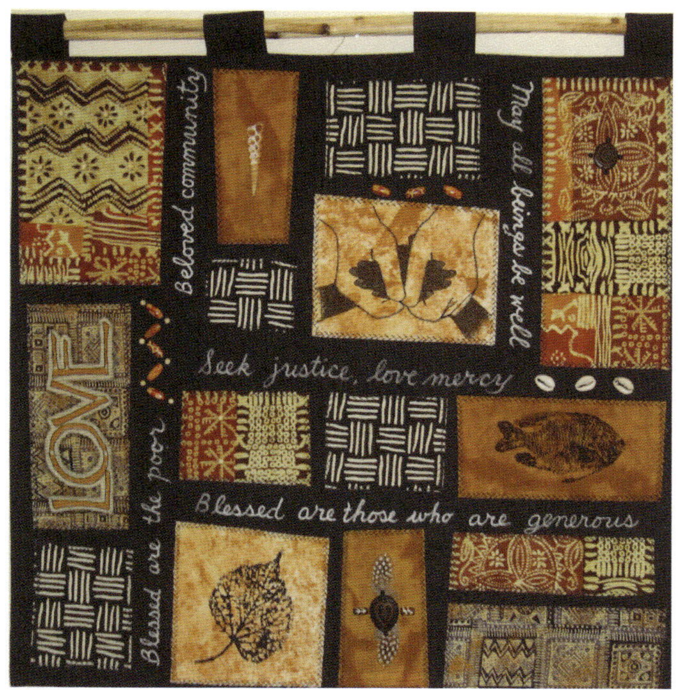

Martha Tabis
Warrenville, IL, USA

Connected
22" x 23"

It's been stated many ways, that we are connected to all of humanity, whether continents away or right in our neighborhood. In the Bantu language our interconnectedness is called "Ubuntu". Martin Luther King described it as the Beloved Community. In Buddhist meditation, the metta "May all beings be well" embodies this spirit. Quotes from scripture printed on this quilt are from Micah 6:8, Proverbs 22:9 and Matthew 5:3. Each speaks of extending compassion to others.

GRIEF

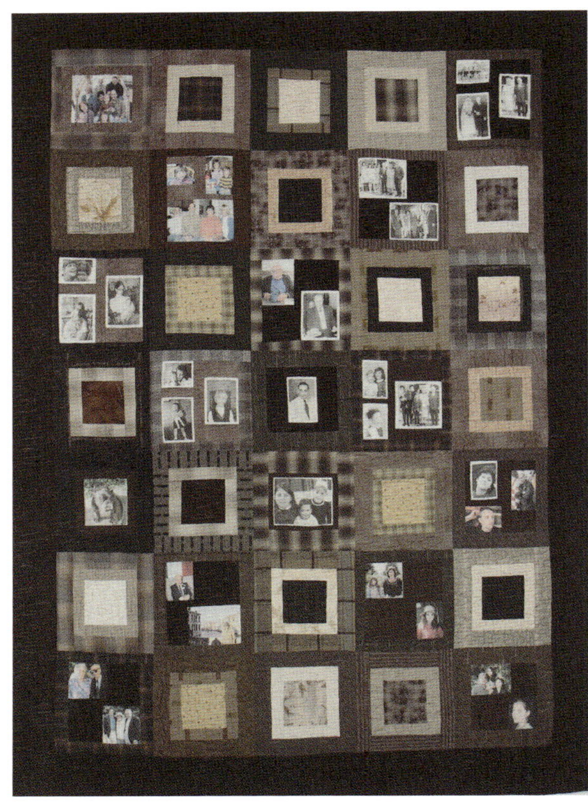

Maxine Foster
Chapel Hill, NC, USA

Dad's Memories
51" x 68.5"

As Alzheimer's slowly destroyed my dad's memories, I was inspired to create a quilt. I wanted it to stimulate his mind and heart with images of family, and as his memories faded, provide him a thing of beauty to delight his eye and calm his gaze. As his life changed dramatically he still occupied the center of the family and those he loved. The quilt is a document of his life and a source of beauty and comfort for someone living without memories. My dad recently died but my memories of him still live on, as does the quilt.

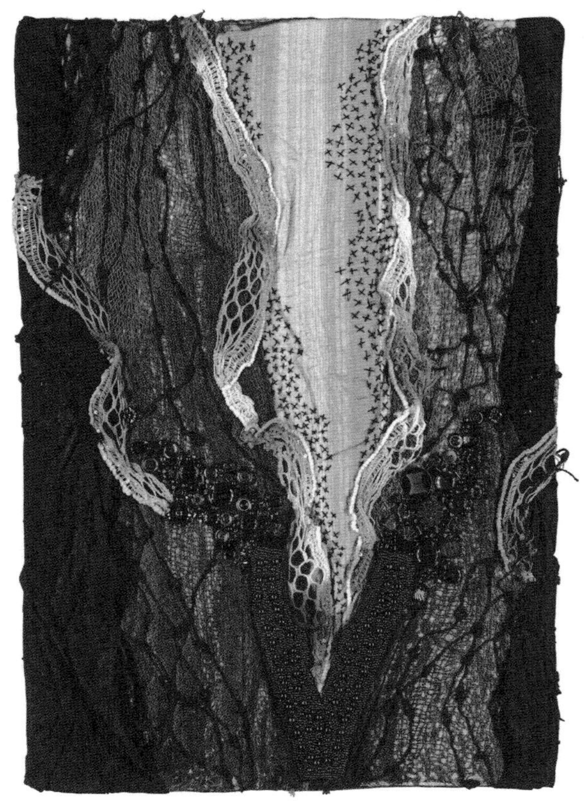

Lisa Quintana Troy, OH, USA
View from the Abyss 23" x 32"

Falling into despondance, grief, despair, and depression, and yet, the light is above, and you an see a way up.

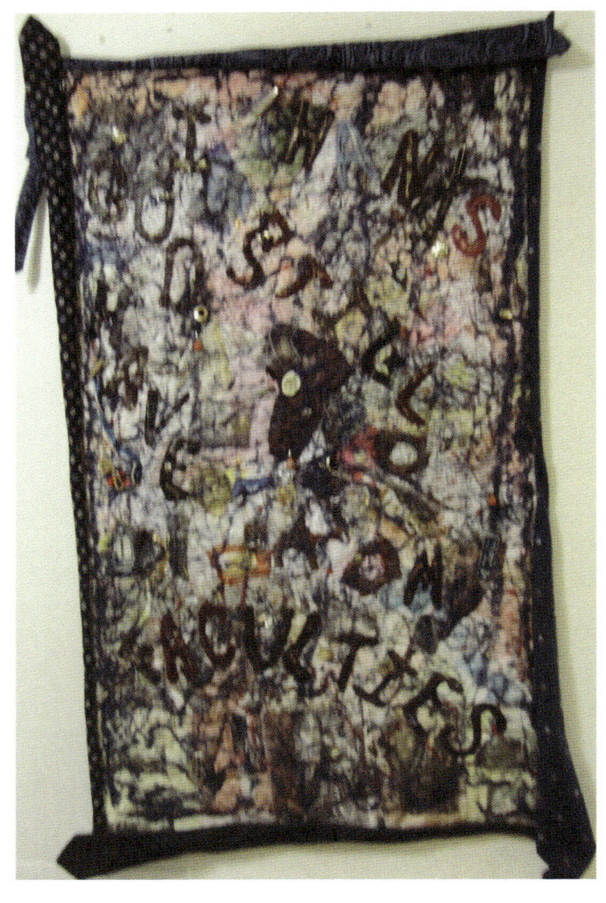

Diana K Shore
Bell Canyon, CA, USA

Lost Memory
33" x 49"

When my father-in-law died of Alzheimer's I wrote on fabric all the phrases that I could remember him saying. I appliqued over and around the words adding old photos of him and his family before many of them perished in the holocaust. I then added some trinkets and keepsakes of his including a namebadge and cufflinks. I stitched one of his speeches on God and creation using water soluable stabilizer. When I rinsed it the words were gone just like in his memory but the texture of his life remained framed by his old neckties. Vinyl samples remind me of his polymer business with one of his last phrases, "Thank God I still have my faculties."

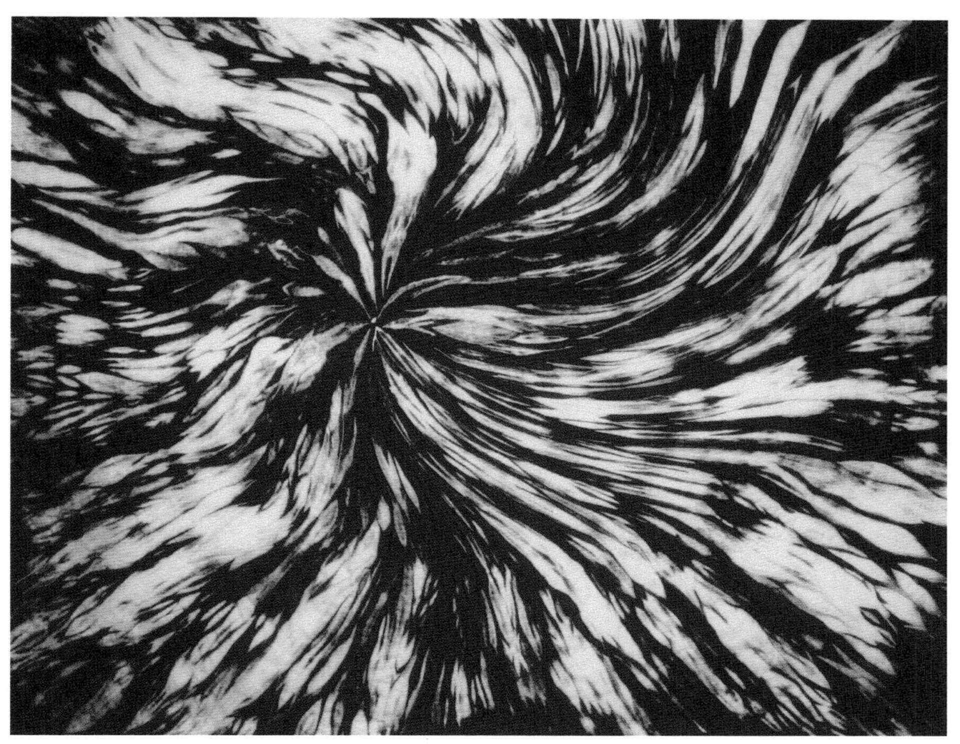

Catherine L Waltz Fort Lauderdale, FL, USA
Maelstrom 41" x 32"

Loss and grief can lead to a maelstrom of despair. After the death of my mother I was very aware of my unstable emotions which came and went in waves over a long period of time. My emotions swirled but there were glimmers of light. This swirling emotional maelstrom threatens to pull one down under but by remaining centered and focused on the glimmers of light one can ride the waves of feeling. I eventually recovered my balance, like a sailboat riding out a storm. It has taken several years to get an image that matched my visualization of my process.

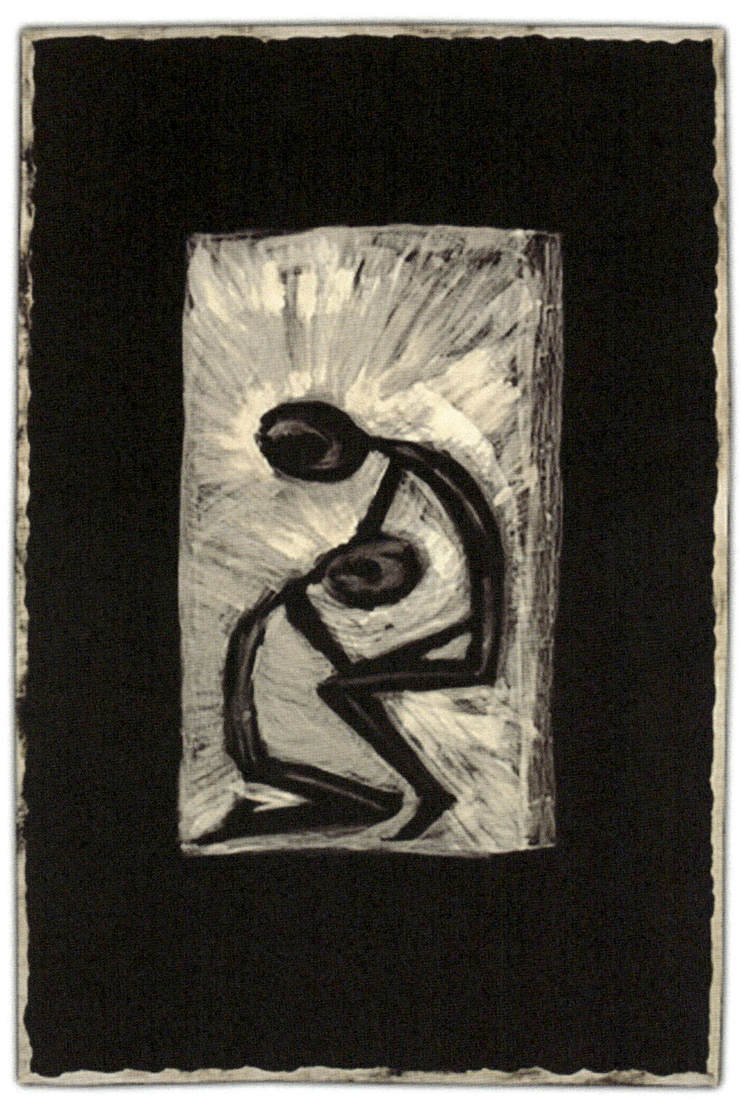

Maggie Weiss
Evanston, IL, USA

Loss
43" x 64"

Losing Patty: Upon arriving home my mother told my father that my big sister Patty had died. Barely inside the door, Dad fell to his knees in shock. Mom cradled him in her lap as they held on to each other in despair. Twenty years later I found a way to portray the vision that was seared upon my heart that cold December night.

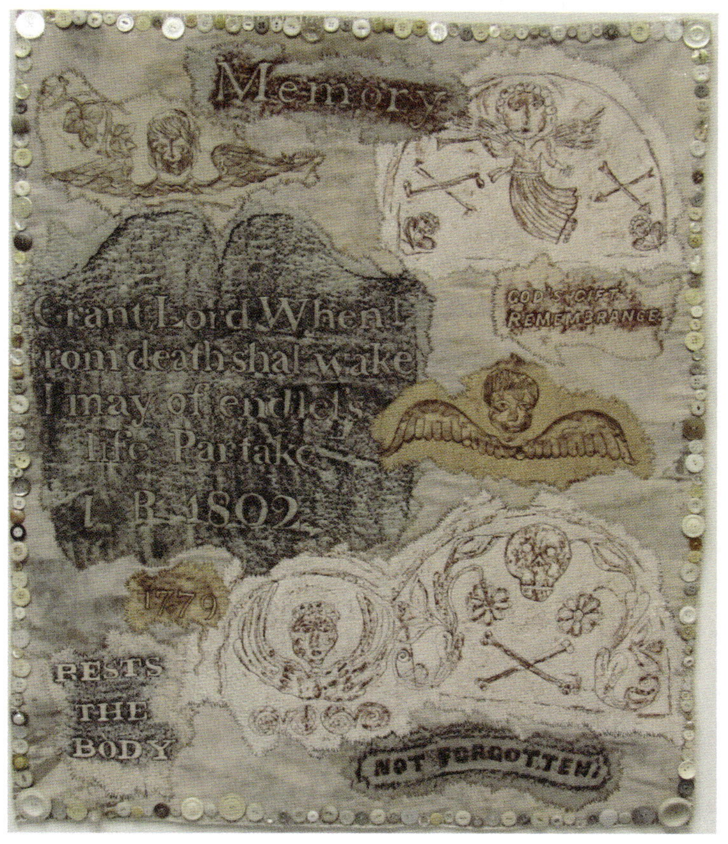

Susan Lenz
Columbia, SC, USA

Endless Life
33” x 38”

Grave rubbings on silk, vintage household linens, recycled material and stitches are meant to reflect both personal and universal mortality and the passage of time through generations. The exploration of final words marking others' lives causes reflection of ones own existence. The work investigates the concept of remembrance, personal legacy, and our common human frailty.

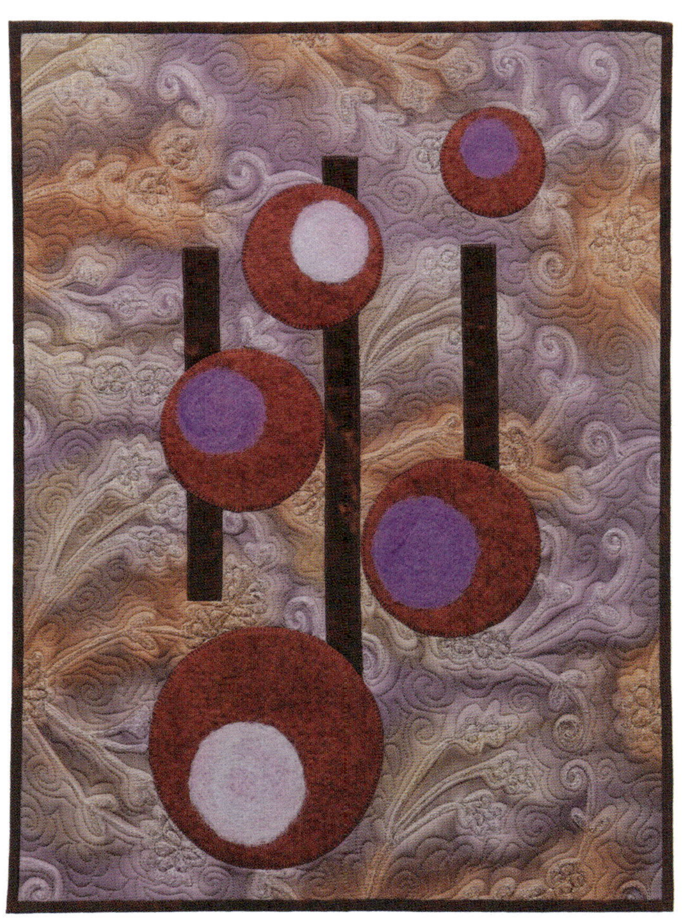

Casey Puetz
Waukesha, WI, USA

Early Mourning
18.5" x 24.5"

A challenge was issued to use a common household item as inspiration for an art quilt. The original color palette for a plastic spatula was too bright, like eggs over easy. However, Mom became seriously ill and the tones took on the sense of mourning for her impending passing.

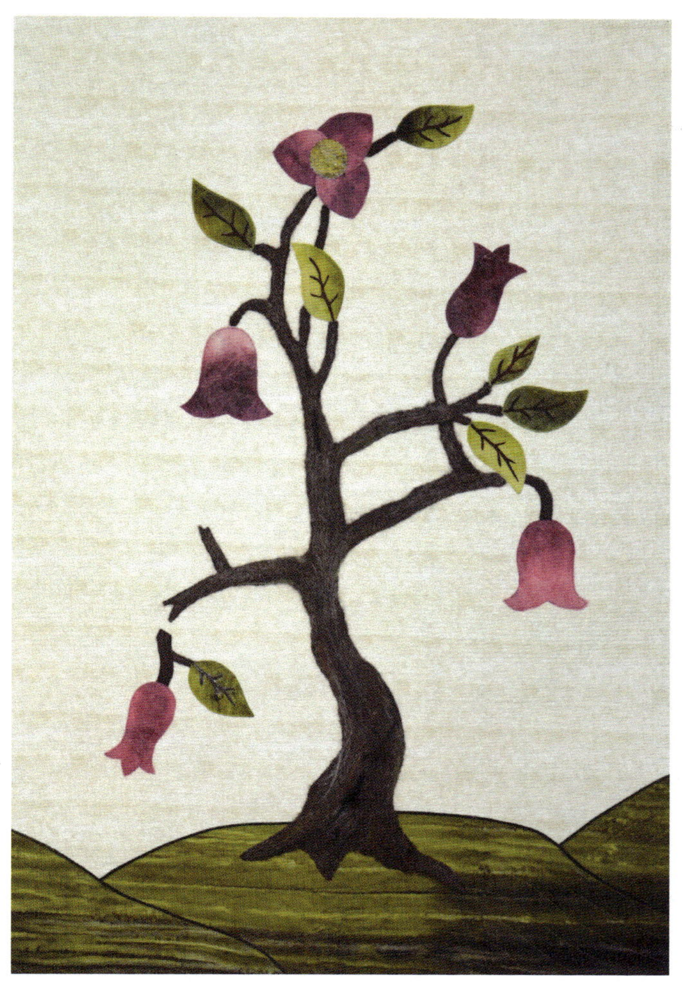

Helen Turnbull
Broad Run, VA, USA

The Broken Branch
30.5" x 43"

This tree represents my family. The broken branch symbolizes my daughter who died after a motorcycle accident. Frances was not only a loving daughter, but a wife, mother, and sister. She was always willing to take time out of her busy day to make time for others. She was an artist who loved to make both quilts and glass work. Frances was a generous person who believed in charity and helping others. She made many quilts for homeless shelters and cancer patients. Frances brought lots of joy to our family and is deeply missed.

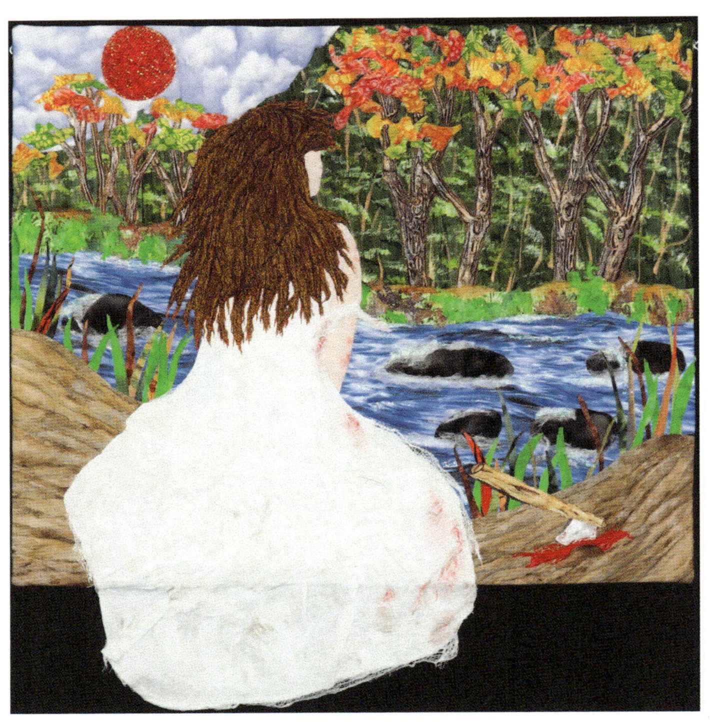

Janice M Jones
Methuen, MA, USA

Hannah Dustin's Revenge
24" x 24"

Hannah Dustin was a colonial Massachusetts Puritan who was taken captive and held hostage by Abenaki Indians. The Abenaki savagely killed her newborn infant before her eyes. During captivity, she and two other English captives used tomahawks to kill and scalp ten of the Abenakis and escaped. There is controversy regarding her actions, but it is established that she was a strong and courageous woman for her time. The focus of my piece is to imagine how she felt in the aftermath of her revenge--after her rage subsided. She is left alone to overcome her grief.

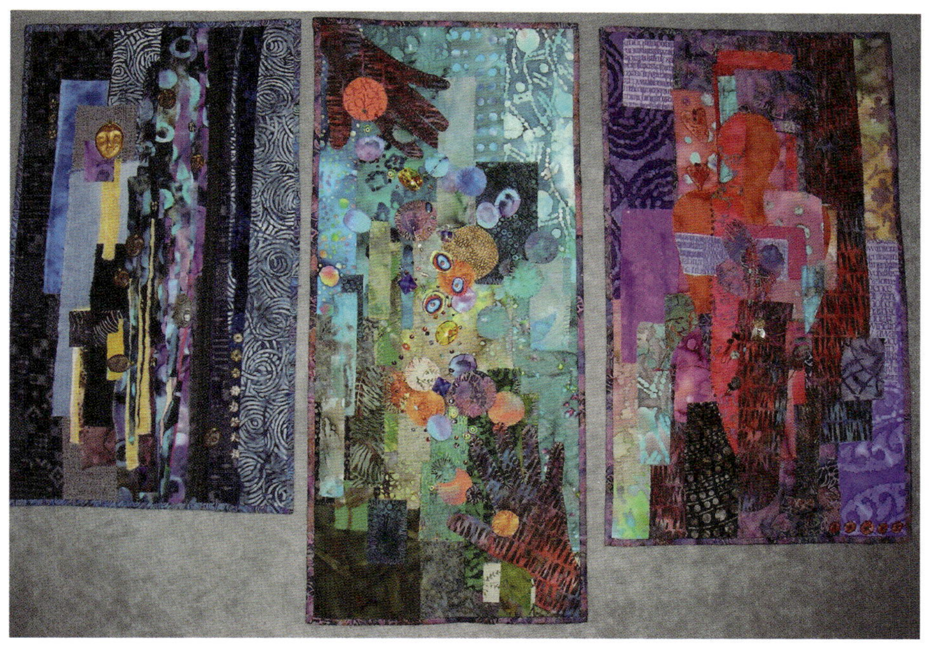

Barbara L Wester Naperville, IL, USA
Loss, Longing, Remembrance 46" x 31"

This quilt symbolizes the journey of my grieving for the loss in a tragic traffic accident of my friend Polly Ullrich. Polly was an artist and art critic, a loving wife and mom. In less than a moment, her life ended after her car was hit by another driver. This quilt takes us through the journey I think all of us travel in coming to terms with death: loss (focusing on the raw absence of someone as a physical presence (face)), longing (focusing on hands reaching and wanting to grasp), and finally remembrance (finding our loved ones in our hearts).

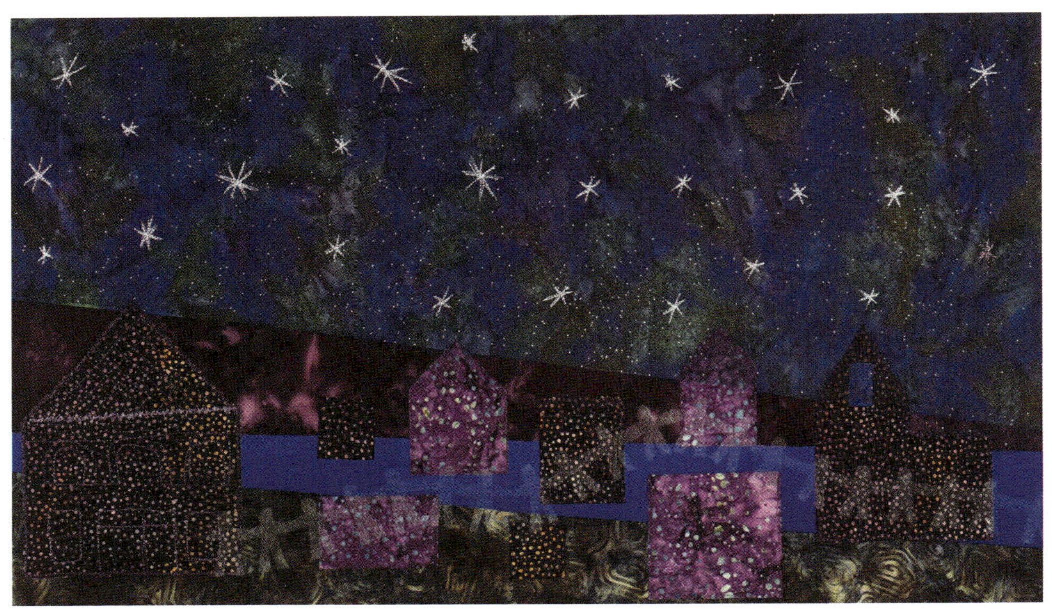

Charlotte Jackson Fort Collins, CO, USA

28 New Stars, One Hidden in Disbelief, One Fallen in Disgrace

27" x 15.75"

Sometimes grief needs a place to go so that healing can follow, for all who were affected, and thus this quilt was born. The tragedy at Sandy Hook school is unspeakable, heartbreaking, incomprehensible and will always be with us. How is it then possible to forgive, when the act is so horrific and so deeply violates society's norms? As a parent, grandparent and retired educator, could I walk the path to forgiveness and compassion, or remain in anger and judgment. This quilt has helped me along that road, and in the process, to remember that there is always beauty and light in the birth of a new star.

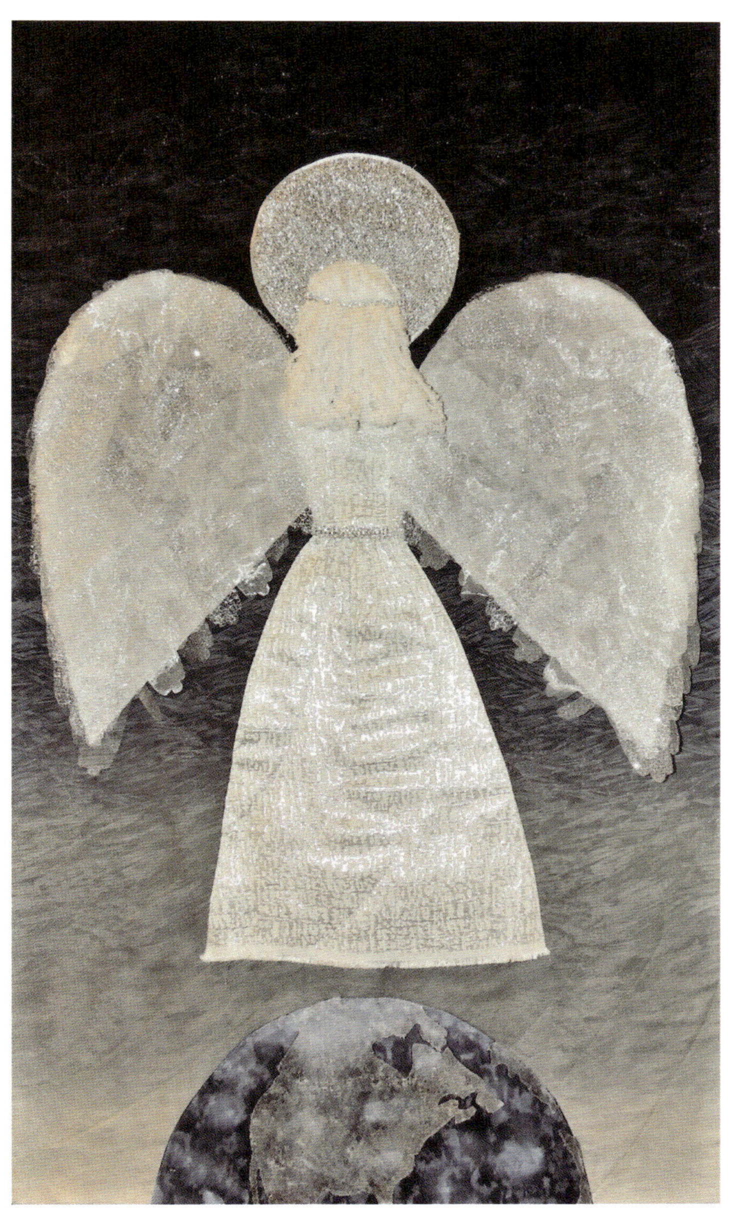

Judi L Shipley
Gig Harbor, WA, USA

Angel of Deliverance
25” x 40”

Twenty children died December 2012 at Sandy Hook Elementary School, Newtown, Connecticut. To honor their memory and to aid in my grief over this senseless violence I imagined an angel delivering their souls into the hands of our Heavenly Father.

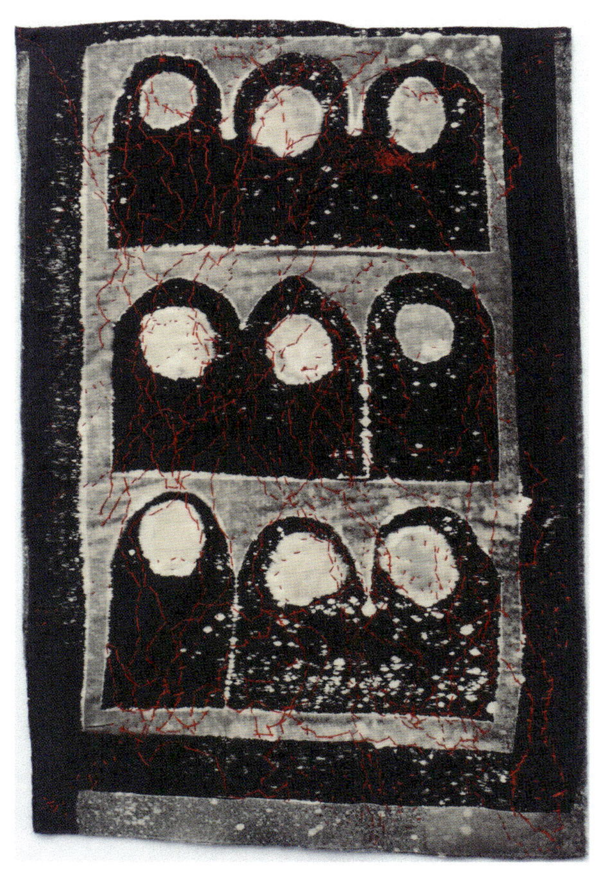

Paula J Swett Lewisburg, PA, USA
There Are No Words 17.5 " x 24.5"

Malala, Gul, Sandy Hook and all unrecognized victims of violence, I have no words. I connect to all of you with my thread and stitches to honor you,your stories and to mark a time when hearts can heal and souls can mend.

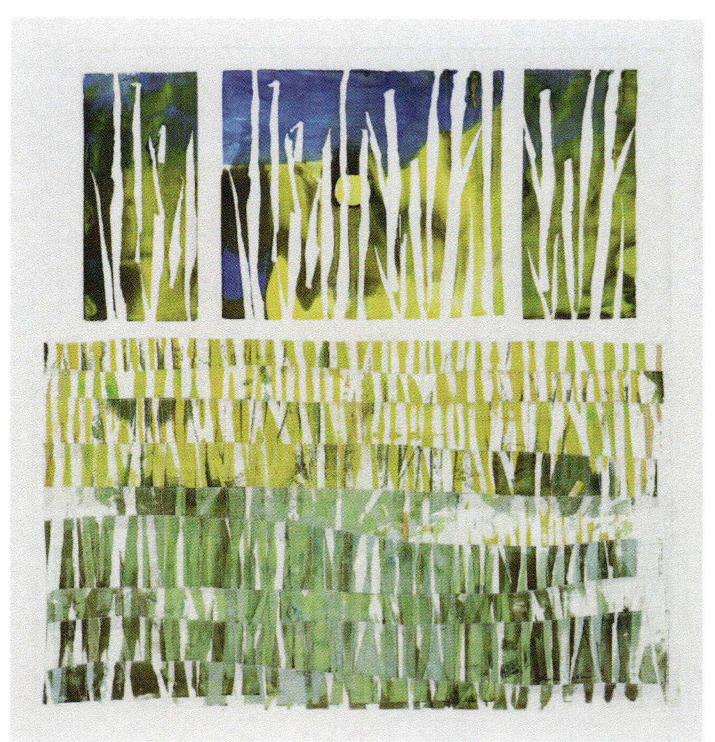

Sharon C Collins Arnprior, Ontario, Canada
Winter Came Too Soon 27" x 27"

This piece was inspired by seeing snow on fields that were still green and not yet ready to reap. I see this as a metaphor of premature death and the sadness of unfulfilled dreams. Memories of our loved ones are frozen at that point never to age.

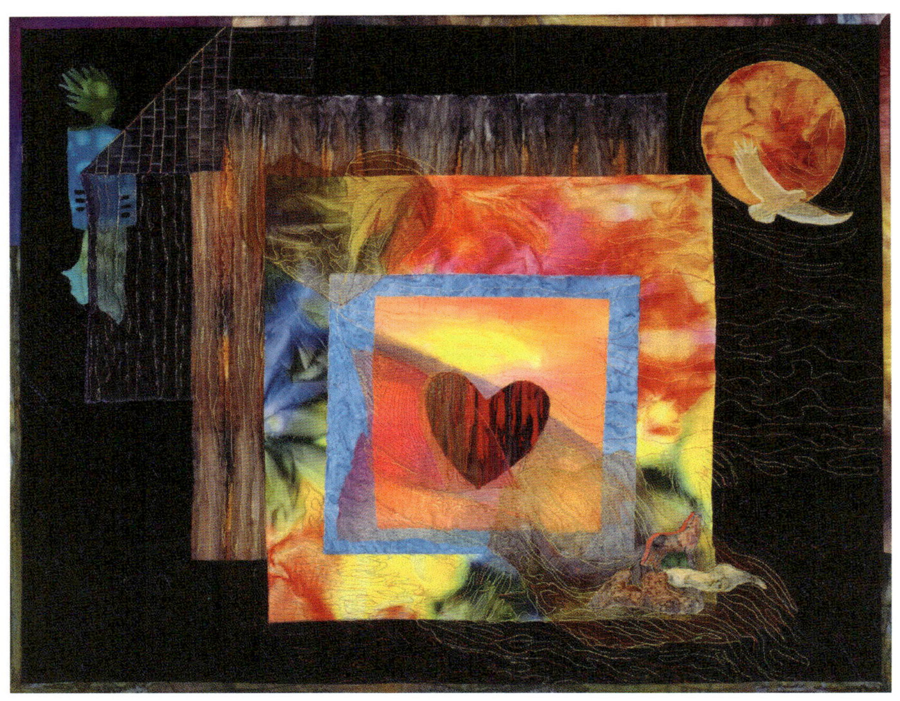

Lyn Wolf Jackson Billings, MT, USA
Joy In the Morning 40.5" x 30"

When he died she lost her tether to earth. Her house and heart darkened until the silvery glimmer of light reflected off her tears. When she sought the Source, she did not grieve as one who had no hope. The howling wolf of grief looked at the Light, did his job, and moved on.

Psalm 30:5 Weeping may remain for a night, but rejoicing comes in the morning.

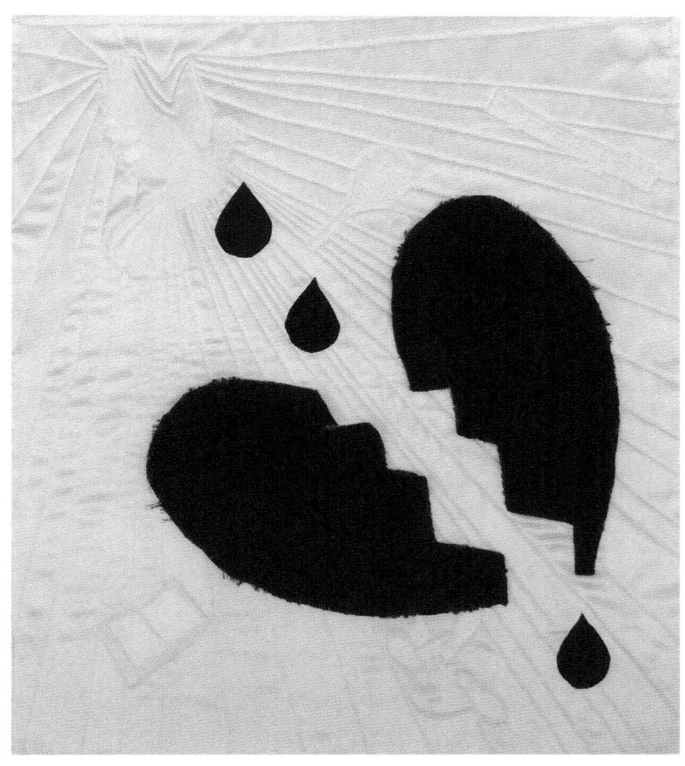

Diane M Schultheiss
Atlanta, GA, USA

Jesus Wept: John 11:35
20.25" x 22.25"

On June 18, 2012, when my husband, Steve Sparkes', heart took its last beat, my heart broke and the color left my world. Through the three months of intensive care God was with us and saved his life many times. I know God is still surrounding us in our time of deep sorrow. This verse has been comforting to know Christ knows our sorrow. The embroidered images represent the things Steve loved doing - playing tennis, reading, singing in his beautiful tenor voice and dancing.

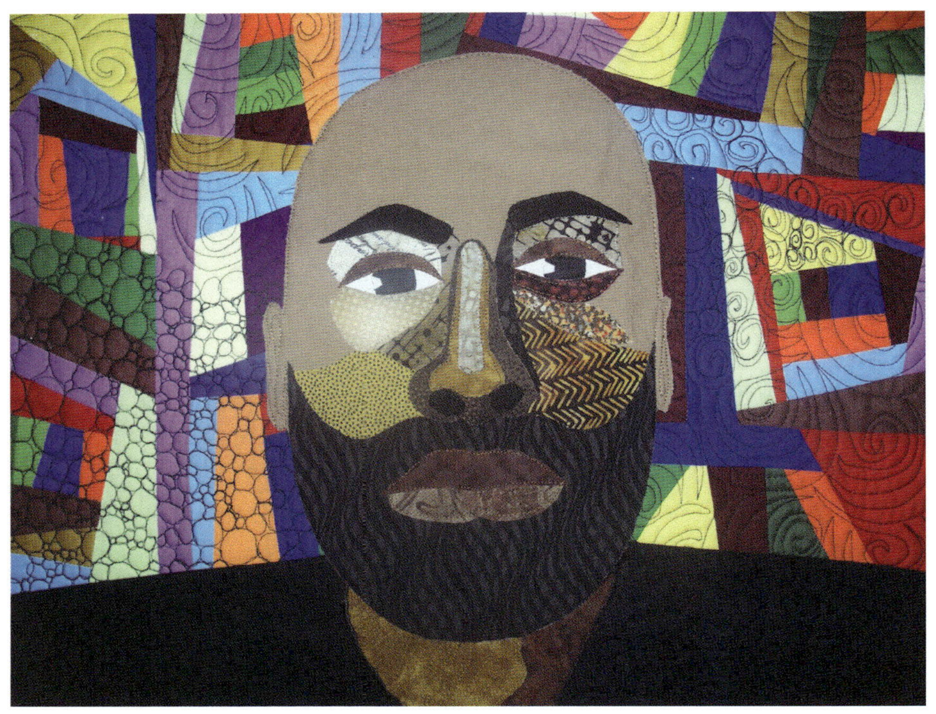

Cheryl D Hurd Washington, DC, USA
Bubba 20" x 27"

Dear Bubba,
You are with us in every moment and in every thought. We feel your love for us all every day - your family, your children, your friends, and anyone who knows you. We hear your words of wisdom, your laughter, your humor. We miss that beautiful smile, your gratitude, humility and generosity. You are a gift from God to us all.
Love, Mom

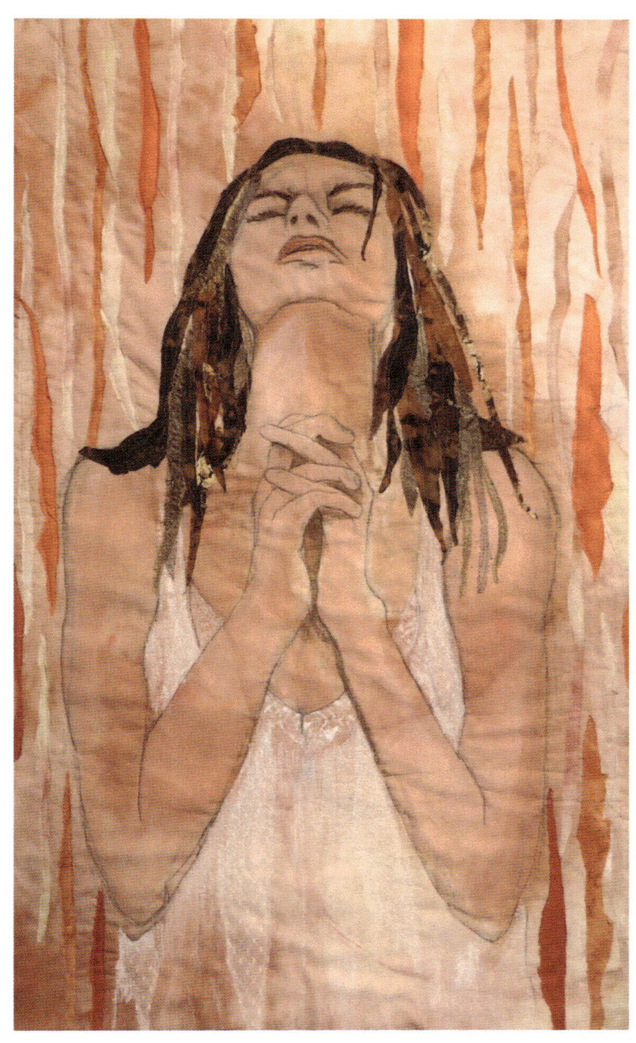

Sharon Tesser
Lawrenceburg, IN, USA

Stages of Grief
21" x 32"

Grief is a multi-faceted emotion. The quilt depicts a moment in time experiencing the pain, loss, and depth of grief. The background is the surprise element to grief; painful slices that appear without warning and cut into the soul. Grief is an emotion experienced by all. I have been surprised by how painful and shocking the moments are when in the midst of an ordinary day I can be overtaken by unexpected waves of grief. It is through the loss of loved ones that I have experienced the weight of grief. I don't know when the process ends.

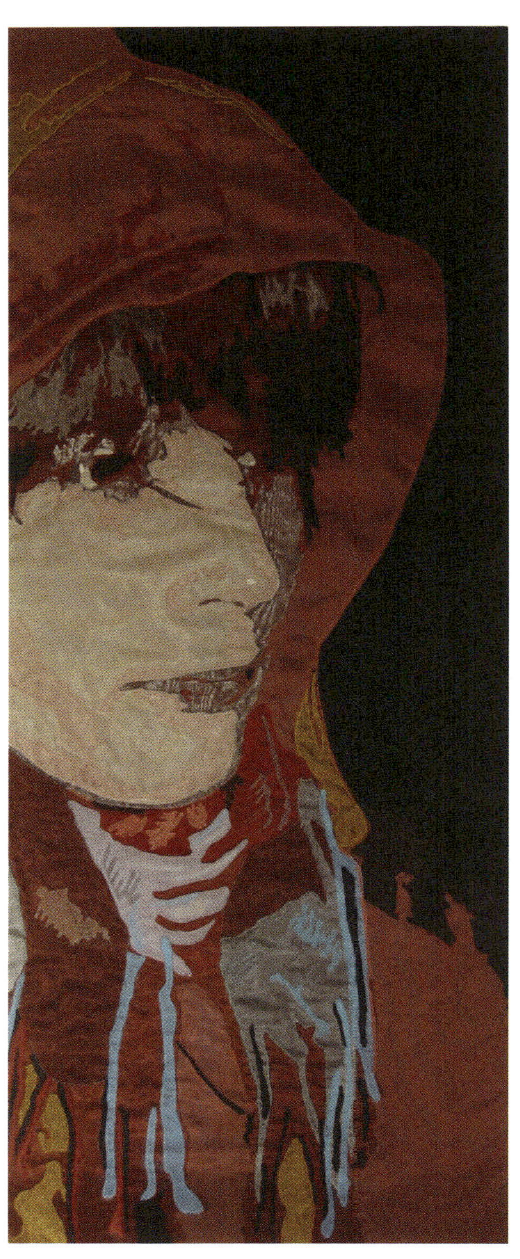

Martha Wolfe
Davis, CA, USA

Just Harry
18" x 45"

adolescent depression
carefree child/paralyzed young adult
darkest hours...
dancing the edge of suicide.
watch the suffering,
helpless to relieve the pain,
the heart reels.

let go...
time, support of many,
a path out of the darkness.
travel together,
different destinations.
take nothing for granted.
each day, a gift.

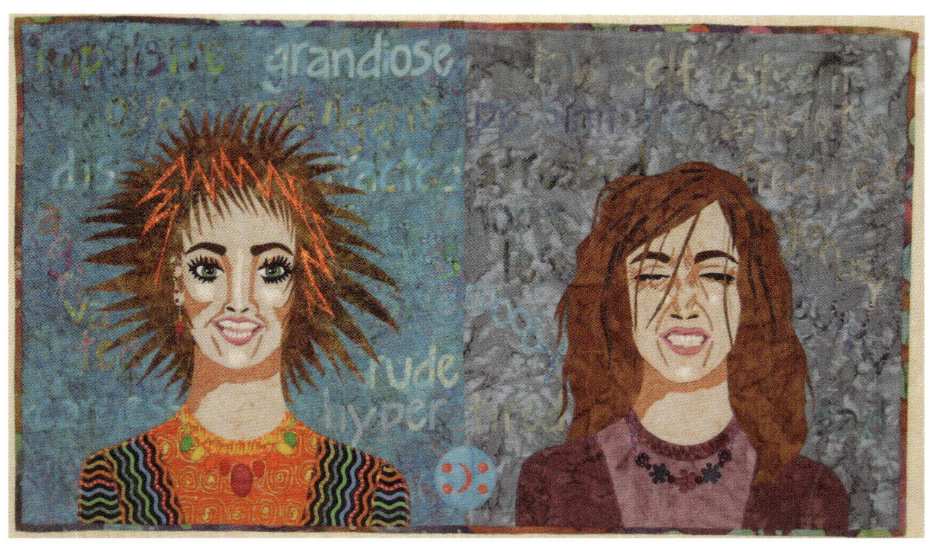

Laurie Ceesay Menominee, MI, USA
My Friend is Bipolar 43.5" x 24.25"

My significant other has Bipolar Disorder. I made this quilt to explore the characteristics of being bipolar, as the person who lives and interacts daily with the mood swings of being manic one day/minute and then depressed the next. I used many descriptive words in the quilt background but purposely made the colors blend because it is symbolic of the social stigma of not discussing mental health issues. I exagerated the manic characteristics of overdoing things-the woman's hair, make-up, jewelry and clothing patterns and colors. With the depressed representation I kept the colors greyed, sad and subdued, the jewelry dark, and the clothing nondescript. I added the universal symbol for Bipolar Disorder in the quilt. My significant other is male but I changed the person in my quilt to a woman for anonymity.

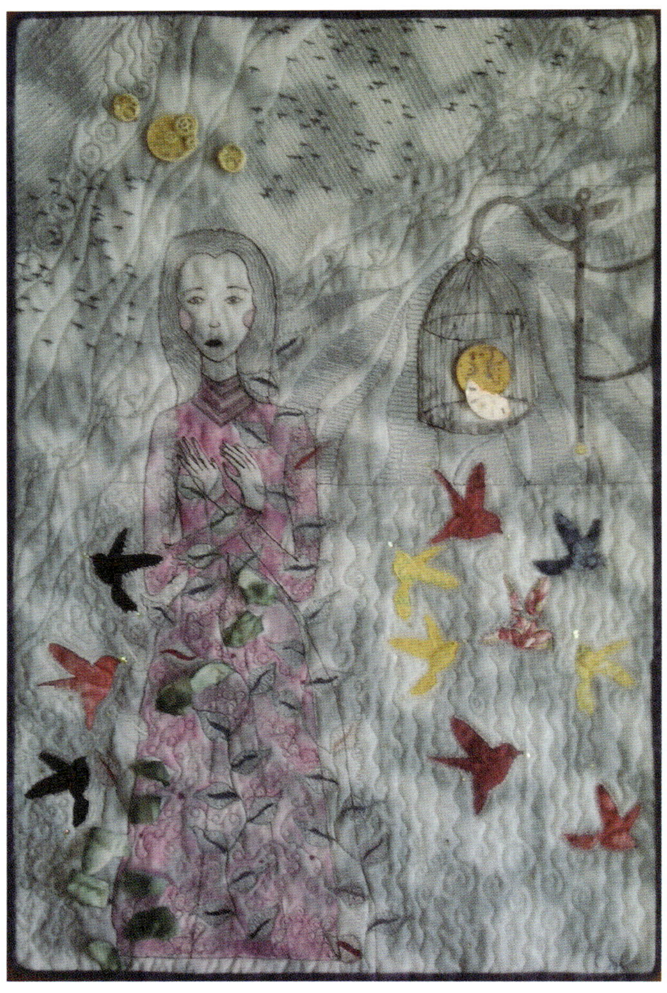

Christine S Cetrulo
Lexington, KY, USA

Depression Series:
3, Frozen
21.5" x 31.5"

Did you ever truly not know WHAT TO DO? Were you frozen by depression? Time stops; loved ones lost. I was so still that my only movement was into a stare, my hands locked in a sad embrace. I was so en-caged, rooted to my sadness that I felt the earth covering me with vines. "Frozen" is a type of memorial to my passed emotions. I look at it now almost wondering who sewed it. My spirit is so far away from her now.
Based on Audrey Niffenegger's aquatint zinc plates - with permission.

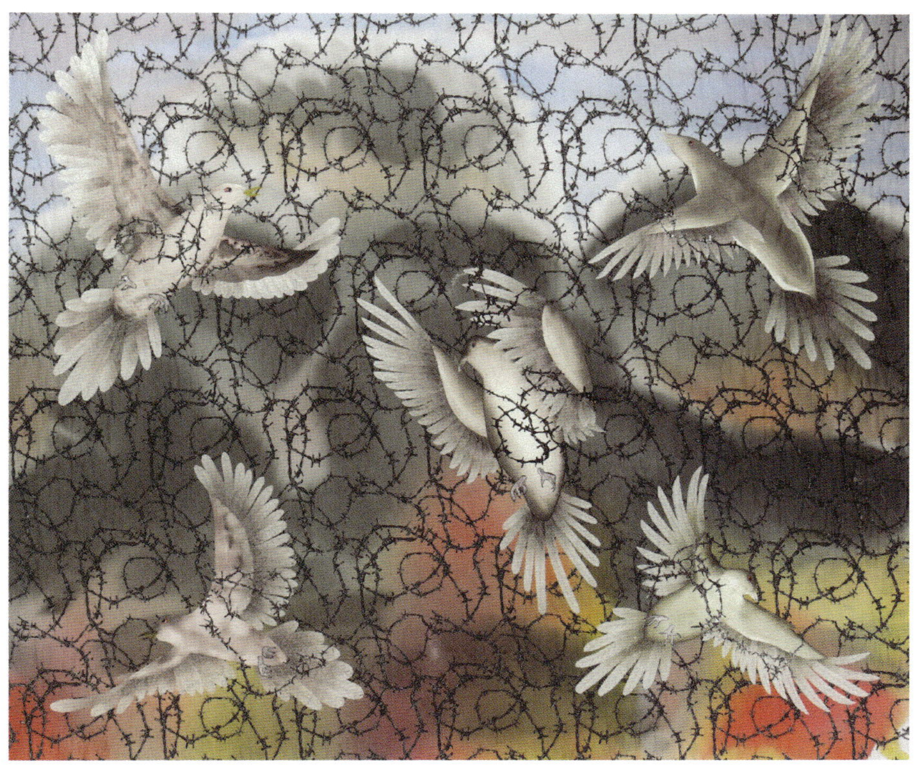

Betty Busby Albuquerque, NM, USA
Mourning Doves 50" x 41"

Even the innocent are caught by the flames of violence and war. Our exchange student from Gaza told us the ways his parents, both doctors, lives have been impacted by continued strife. That was the inspiration for this piece.

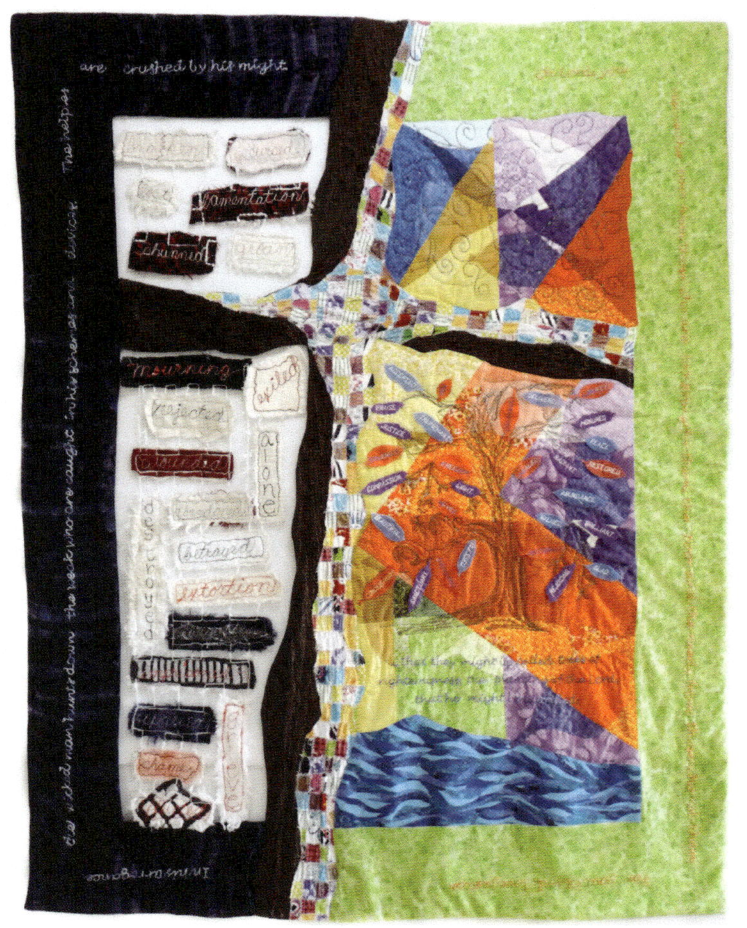

Beverly Manual
Indianapolis, IN, USA

Justice Restored
38.5 x 48

This is my first attempt at making an art quilt. I am involved in anti-human trafficking endeavors in my city of Indianapolis, which is the theme of my quilt. I wanted to depict the transformation that can take place in the life of a trafficked victim through counseling and the work of God in their life after they are rescued. The checkered section of the quilt is scrap fabric used by rescued and restored girls in Cambodia to make accessory items they sell to support themselves. The organization is Sak Saum in Phnom Penh, Cambodia.

FOREVER
DONT WORRY MAMA
ILL TAKE CARE OF YOU
ILL NEVER BREAK YOUR HEART
GROW OLD WITH ME...THE BEST IS YET TO BE
ITS PROBABLY NOTHING
NEXT YEAR

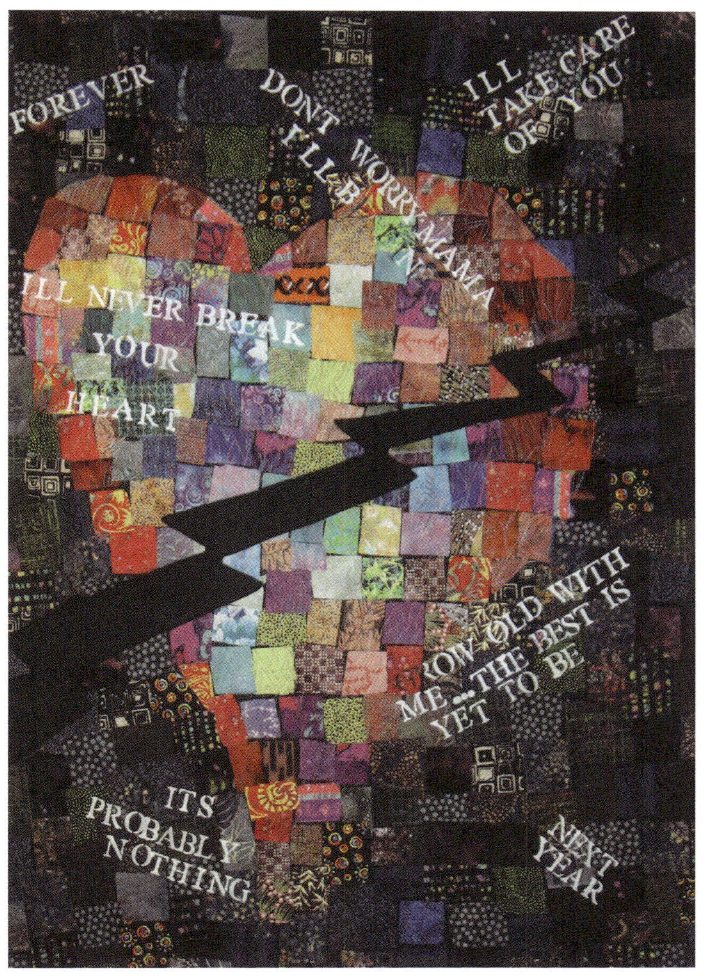

Merrilee J Tieche
Nixa, MO, USA

Broken Promises
34" x 46"

Just before he died unexpectly, my dear husband gave me a sundial inscribed with the phrase, "Grow Old With Me - the Best is Yet to Be". That would never happen. A few years after that my beloved daughter, my only child, was diagnosed with ovarian cancer at age 34. She lived five very difficult years after that. So many things they had both said stayed with me, fueling my anger at the injustice of it all. Making this quilt put a face to my grief and allowed a dialog with my subconscious. The healing process is on-going.

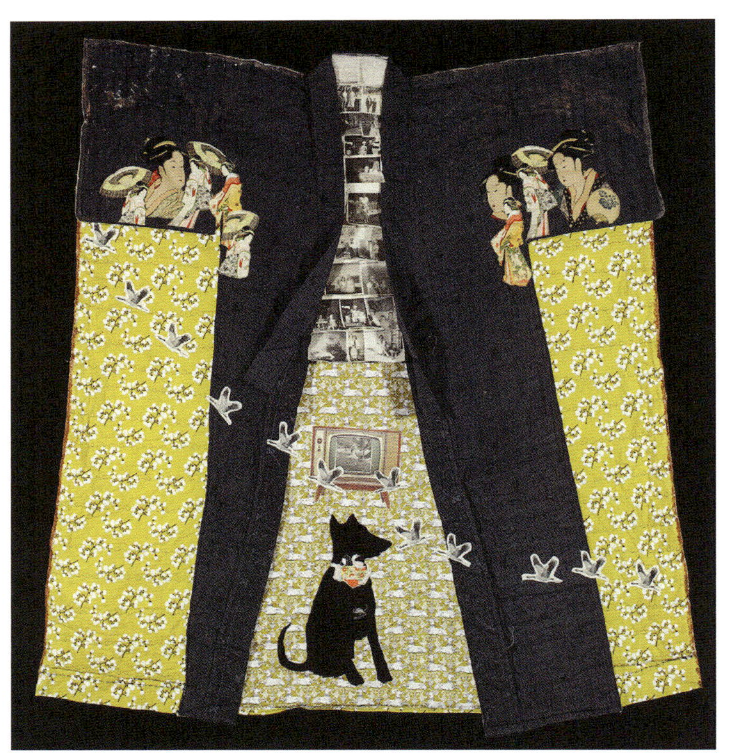

Margaret Abramshe Arvada, CO, USA
The Souls That I Pray To 48" x 56"

This quilt is shrine to members of my family who have died or drifted away from me. A kimono opens up as a symbol of my inner life. Inside the lapels are memories of my childhood contained in old photos of my sister and me with our parents. The opening at the bottom highlights the ghost of my favorite dog gazing at a flock of sacred cranes heading to heaven. Remembering is a prayer to the souls who are not with me. It keeps them alive in the presence of my love.

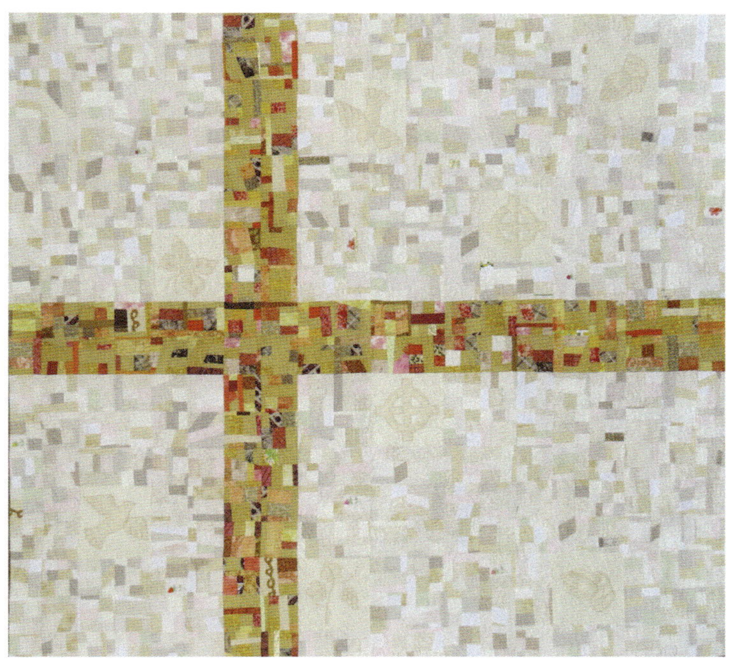

Susan C Clayton Port Orange, FL, USA
Funeral Pall 75" x 78.5"

This is a funeral pall or casket cover for funerals in our sanctuary. For those services without a casket, the pall is hung from a loft. It is made up of over 3000 pieces: bed and table linens, upholstery fabric, garments, lace, vintage, antique and modern fabric submitted by the members of the congregation. The central idea is that in death as in life, Christians are covered by the Body of Christ. As the church, we are the Body of Christ and we uphold the grieving family with our prayers and love.

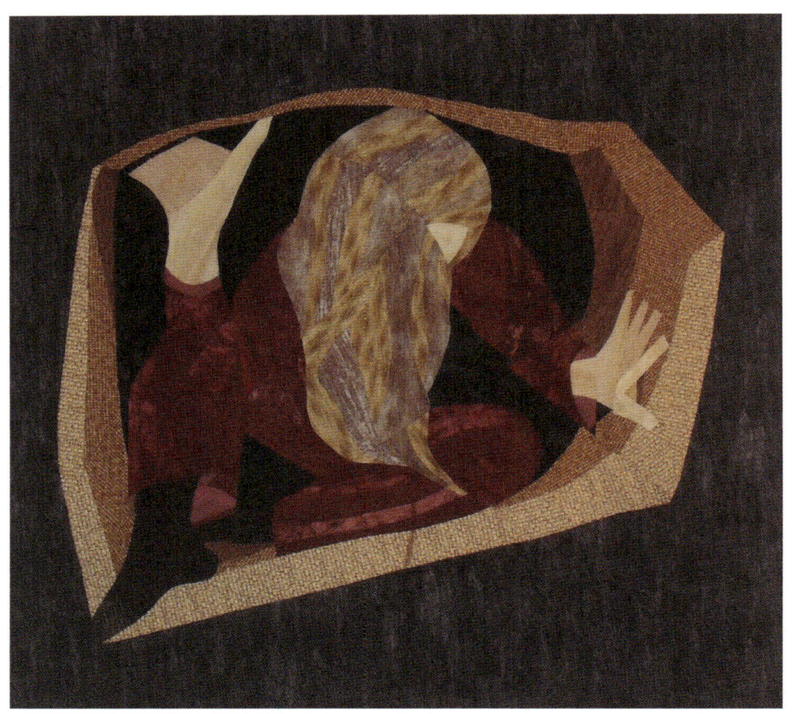

Mary E Simmons Fairfax, VA, USA
Loss and Recovery 38.75" x 34.5"

This image of a lady in a box is my representation of the overwhelming feeling of grief. It portrays the crushing sadness experienced upon the loss of a loved one. Last fall I lost a dear friend. The plans we had made were just not to be. This image also represents the pushing out and away from grief. Recovery is in good memories and trusting in God.

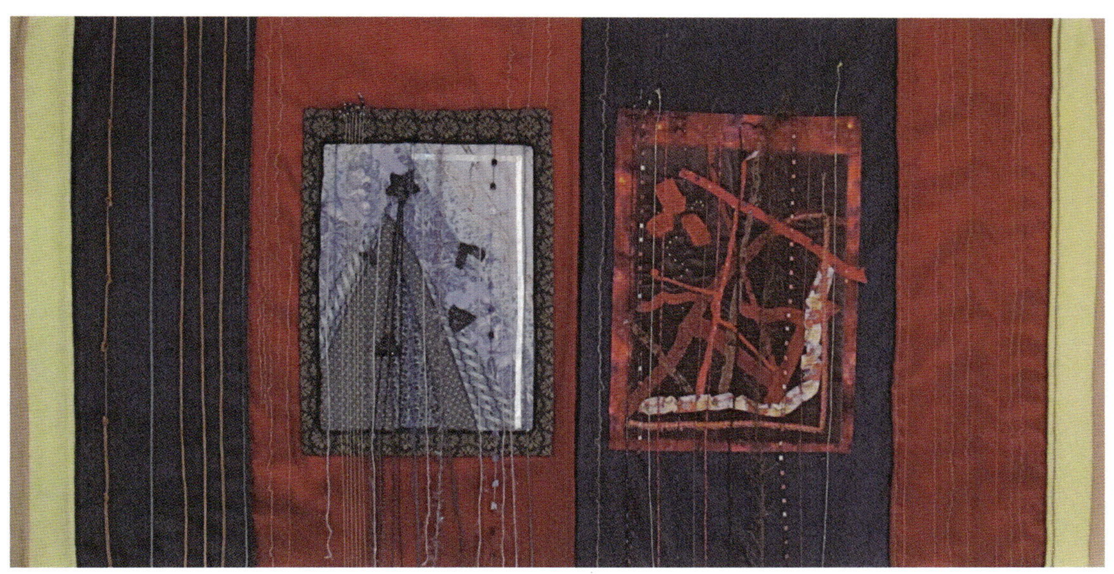

Elaine W Evans Middleburg, VA, USA
String Theory - A Journey of Healing 48" x 24"

Physics string theory - "the universe is quite literally made up of tiny strings" - brought me an "ah ha" moment that has helped me begin to comprehend a 7-year emotional roller coaster ride. My own strings have been tangled, kinked, broken, and frayed. It began with my husband having a "mild" stroke. We've been in denial, anger, depression, resignation, and finally my realizing that the person I knew as my husband is no longer. I need to redefine who and what I am, and establish a new relationship with my life partner. This quilt is my map to moving from grief, through healing, and journey of discovering how my strings are connected, their strengths, and my artistic gifts.

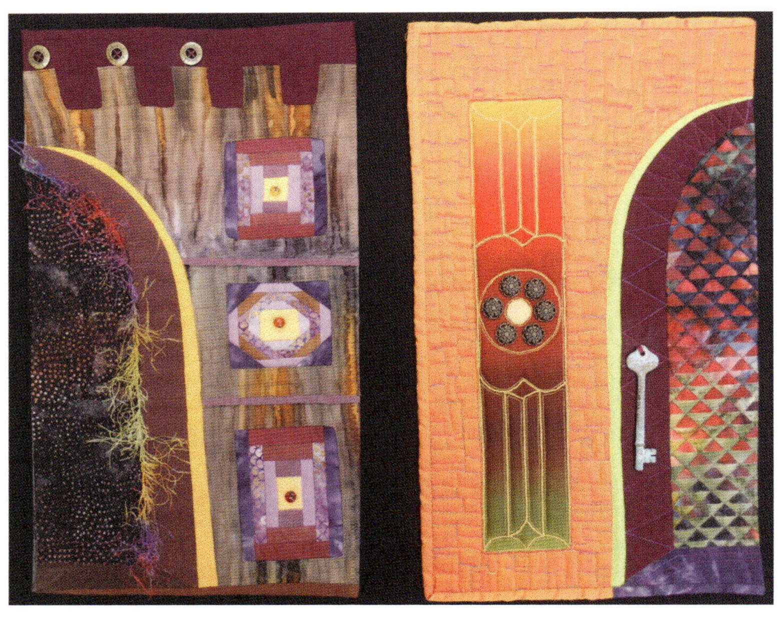

Deborah Sorem Salem, OR, USA

Welcoming Doors: Part one "The Visit", Part two "The Answer"
36” x 28”

I was troubled by my father's decision to move to a state that legalized assisted suicide for the purpose of ending his life even though I was doubtful that he would meet the guidelines. My final decision was to be a supportive and loving daughter and provide him with dignity. While making this quilt I had a flash back to a picture in my Sunday School class room "Jesus Knocking at the Door" and it affected my plans. My quilt evolved into two parts. Their completion brought me a sense of quiet acceptance of my father's decision.

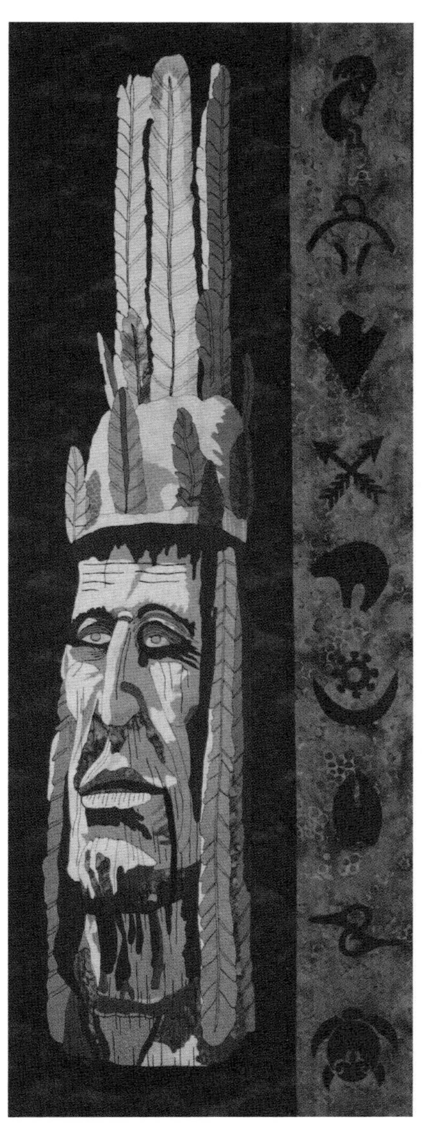

Judith Heyward
Hendersonville, NC, USA

Bearing Witness
22" x 54"

This Indian is part of a wooden statue located at Charlestowne Landing in Charleston, SC. The expression on his face--stoic, sad,strong--is a reminder of all the oppressed people in the world who have died or shed blood because someone else either wanted what they had or for some type of prejudice. The red tear represents this loss and stands as a reminder that we all should "bear witness" to these wrongs and work to eradicate them in the future.

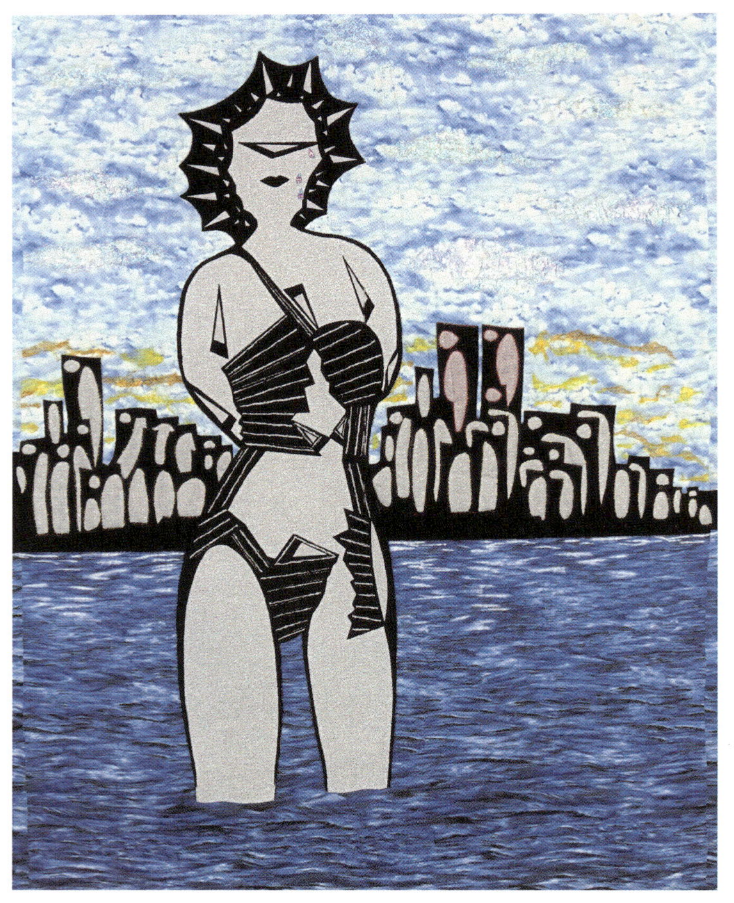

Janice M Jones
Methuen, MA, USA

A Nation Wept
32"x 40"

My father was dying of lung cancer, so I was already grieving when the unspeakable 9/11 attack struck. I was living in New York and the air was thick with grief, shock, fear, and uncertainty. My neighborhood was quiet, and was draped in flags. The heavy atmosphere pushed me to the edge of my personal sorrow. Images of Lady Liberty formed in my mind's eye. She had shed her tears and her robe of grief and was standing strong wearing her battle gear. I felt her battle.

My husband, David Jones, was a key contributor in designing my "Liberty" image.

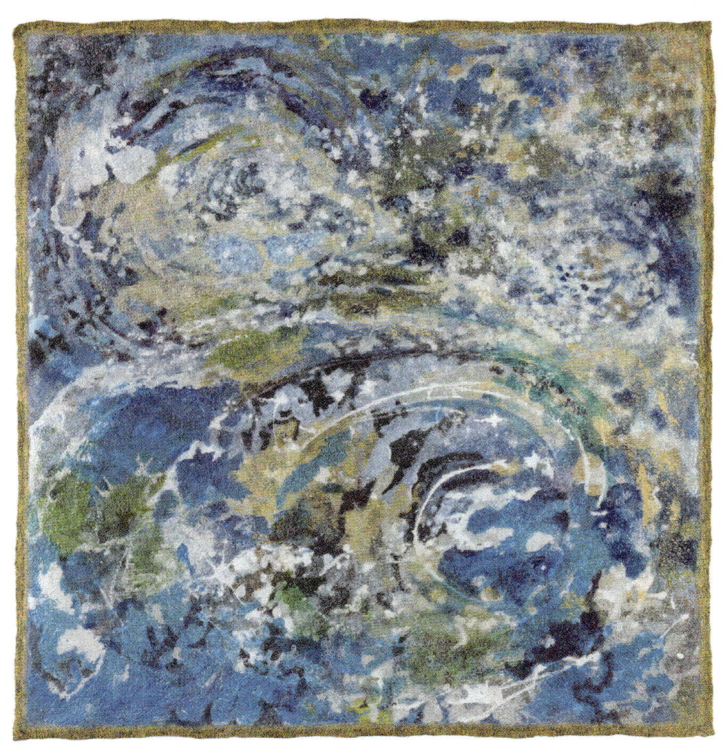

Marianne R Williamson Miami, FL, USA
Pollution in the Gulf 38" x 38"

The oil spill in the Gulf affected me in a deep way because I live and take inspiration for so much of my work here in Florida. The oily, metallic look makes a statement that even though it could be construed as beautiful, it has an unhealthy look.

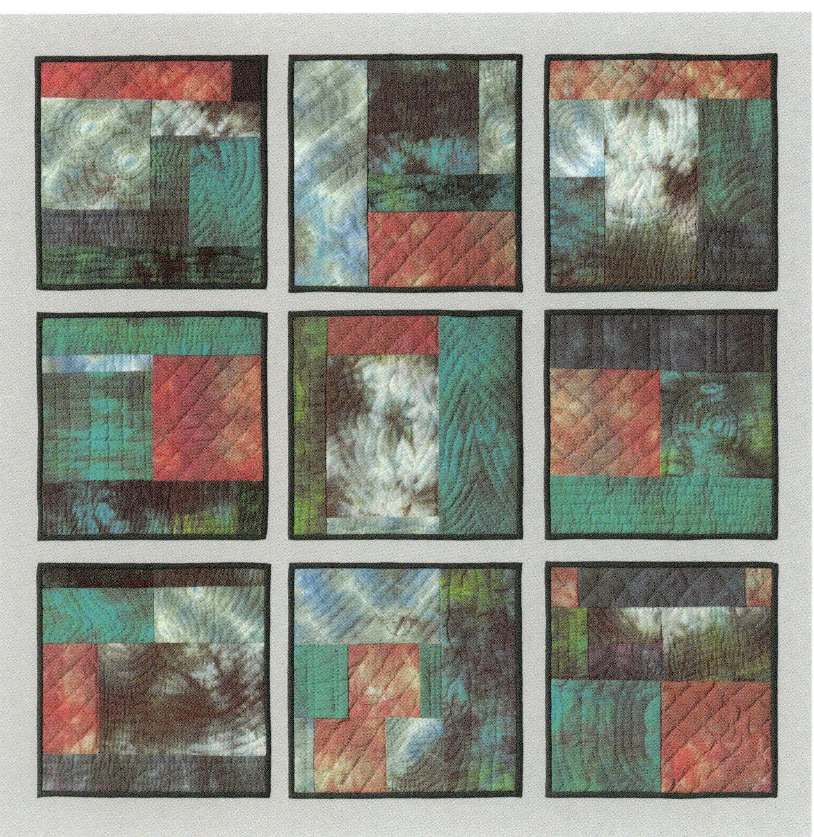

Jill C Le Croissette Carlsbad, CA, USA
Tristesse 38” x 38”

Tristesse is composed of nine tiny quilts expressing my continuing sadness after the death of my husband. The slow process of hand stitching these small pieces brought me a kind of comfort. I live and move in the world, I even smile, but the pain never goes away.

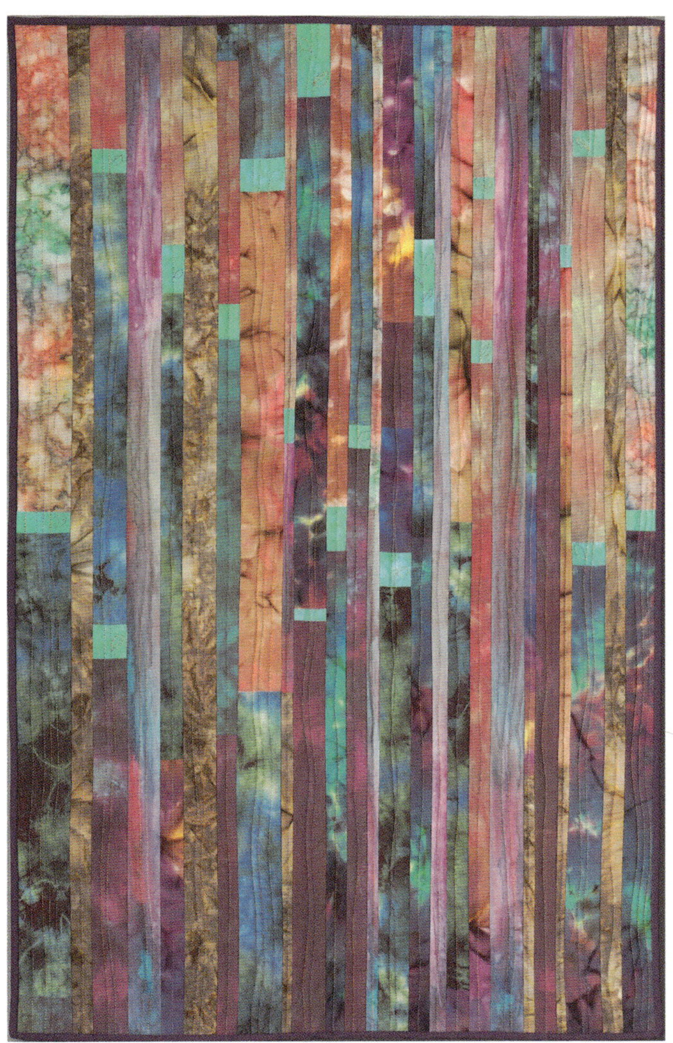

Jill C Le Croissette
Carlsbad, CA, USA

Gleaning (Life Cycles)
28" x 44"

Gleaning is the eighth in my series of Life Cycles quilts, each quilt celebrating a decade of my life. As I reach my 80th year, I feel I am gleaning the precious fragments left after the full harvest has been gathered. The pleasure of remembering good times when my husband was alive helps me through the sadness of facing old age alone.

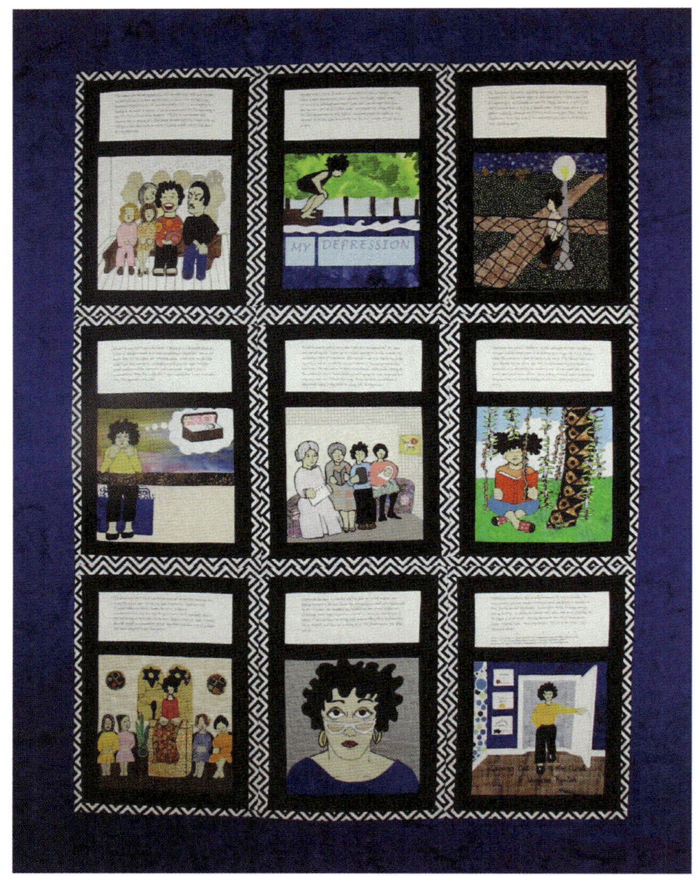

Susan Walen
Bethesda, MD, USA

Not Just Blue
42" x 52"

Depression caused several of my colleagues to suicide. As psychologists, we never spoke about our own depression. They, like me, suffered an illness that was "supposed" to be for others -- not mental health care professionals. We lived in secret, with our own tides of grief, despair, anxiety and self-doubt.

One of the healthiest things I learned to do in my career was to come out of my closet. I gave talks, workshops, wrote papers and a book, and now offer my story-quilt about my journey in owning depression. Perhaps someone will find it helpful.

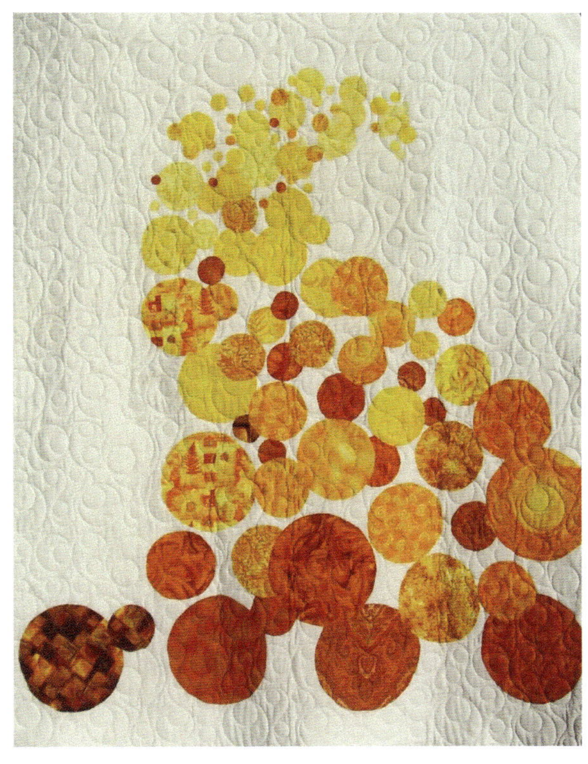

Susan W Ritter
Sierra Vista, AZ, USA

Memories of Mother
60" x 72"

I made the first blue blocks while keeping my ill mother company. When she died suddenly, I finished the remaining blue blocks and called it "Sometimes the Blues." I had never made a quilt without her, and it hung on my design wall for months. Then I realized this wasn't my last thought on the subject. Remembering a line from a Maya Angelou poem, "But still I rise," I made the other side. Dark orange bubbles begin deep within each square, but break free, rising higher and lighter with every turn. I stand mid-stream in generations of quilters -- and still we rise!

Vivien Lemoine, Hereford, AZ, professional quilter

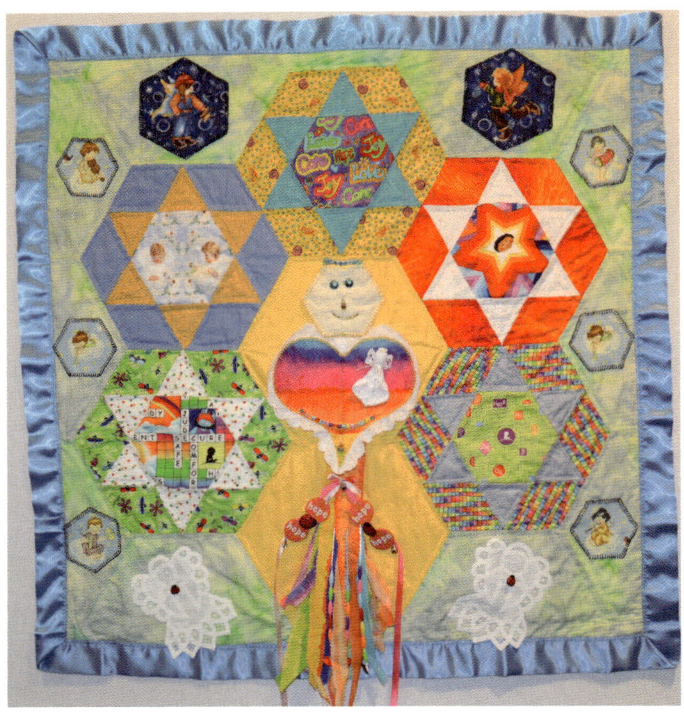

Janet Purlee Jeffersonville, IN, USA

Angel of Hope 36" x 36"

Angel of Hope was created in memory of Hannah Elizabeth Taylor. She lived with and died from childhood cancer. The blocks in this quilt were made in 2004 when I was grieving the loss of my health, the deaths of my Dad and my Brother. The quilt blocks were put away along with my dreams. A Church Quilt Challenge in 2012 brought hope anew. Ladybugs are a universal symbol of Hope. The angel's ragged skirt represents the turmoil and struggle mingled with strings of hope. The satin blanket binding reminds me of the "touchable" nature of all God's angels.

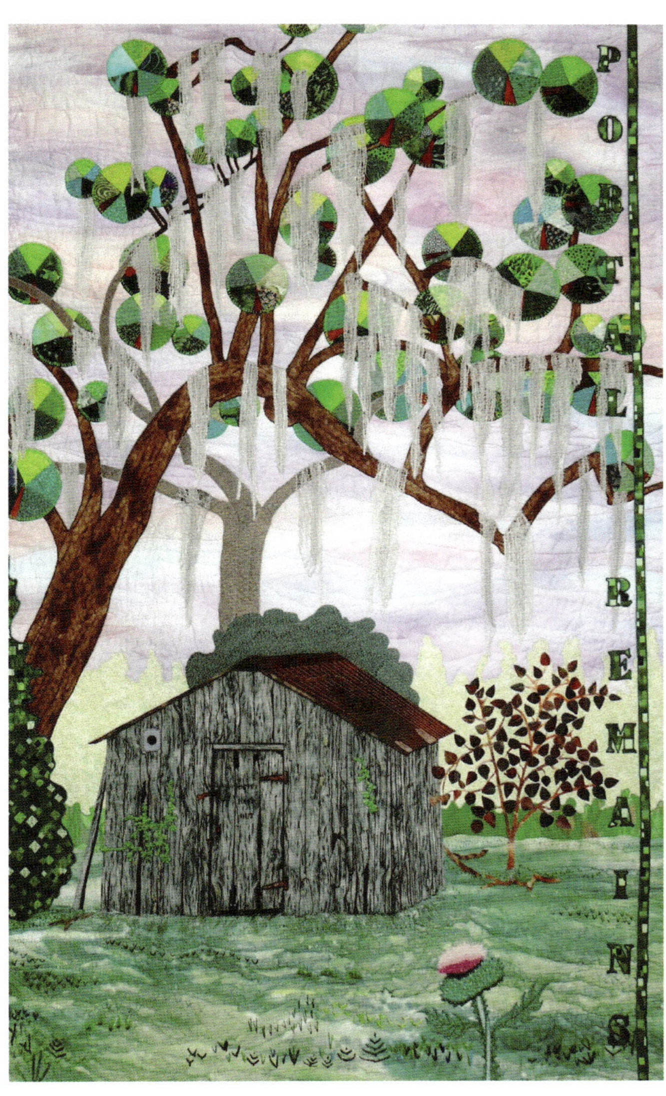

Suzanne M Riggio
Wauwatosa, WI,
USA

Portal Remains
32" x 50"

I grieve at the passing of time. This cypress shed on the banks of Louisiana's Bayou Teche is all that remains of my grandparents' homestead, once vibrant with 7 children, oodles of grandchildren and a well-beaten path to this wash-house door. Now it is weedy, vine ridden, and home to critters, with the shed's door listing on its rusty hinges.

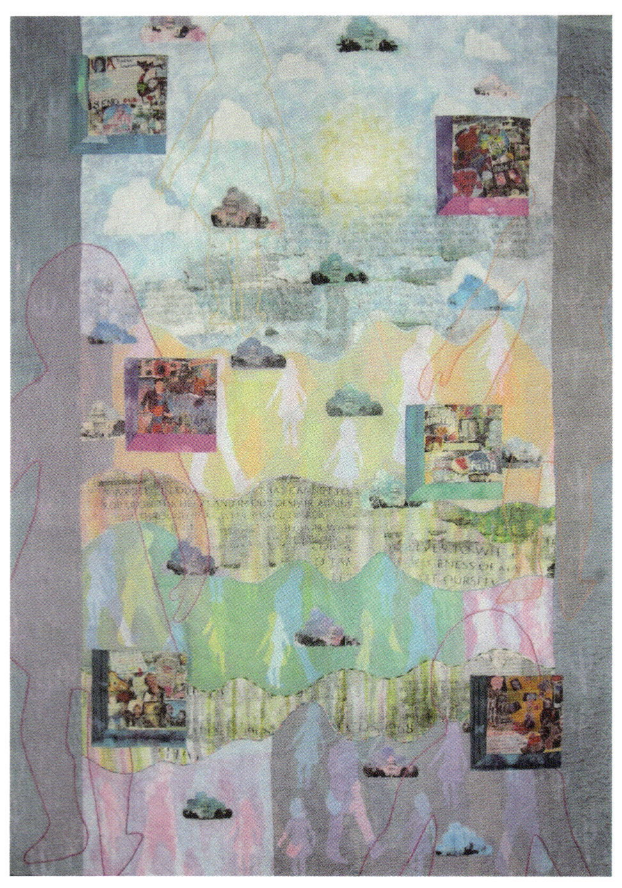

Clare A Aylward
Tucson, AZ, USA

Six Windows
62" x 87"

I'm a quilt artist and social worker in Tucson, Arizona.

January 8, 2011, was warm, sunny. On the radio news of a mass shooting outside a nearby Safeway. Among the dead: a little girl, a judge, a congressional staffer, a retired Republican. The many injured, at a hospital where outside memorials grow daily.

In my quilt, I honor the dead and what is gone forever. I use Robert Kennedy's speech from the day MLK was killled to link past assassinations with the January 8th attempted assassination of Congresswoman Gabrielle Giffords. I ask, when will we stop accepting violence as inevitable in our politics?

HEALING

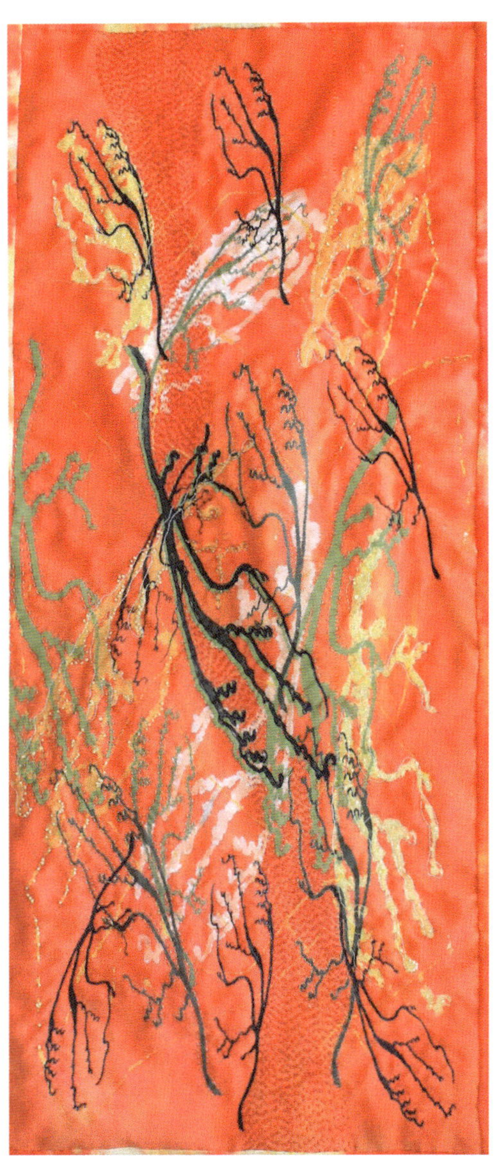

Judy Carpenter
Gainesville, GA, USA

Second Stage
13.75" x 31"

My 94-year-old mother was under Hospice care during the last two weeks of her life. I was overwhelmed with grief, but found solace while working in my dye studio when I was not with Mom. It was too painful to view these pieces after her death, but now almost two years have passed, and I have begun to finish them. This is the first piece.

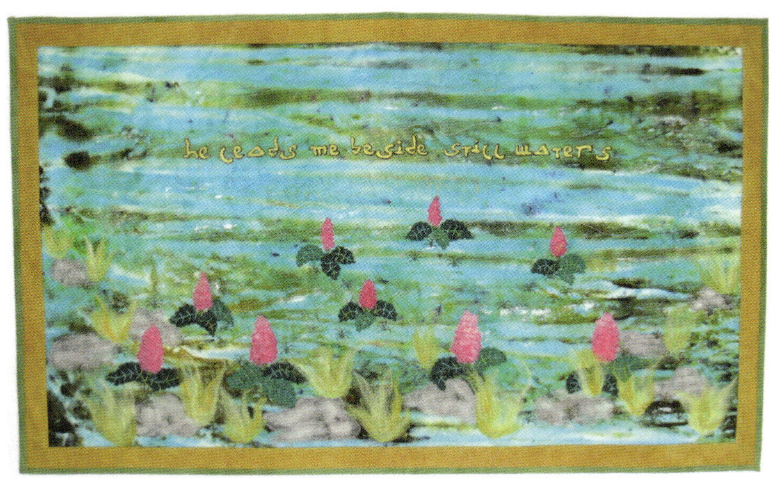

Martha Tabis Warrenville, IL, USA
Beside Still Waters 35" x 21"

In the last months of my mother's life when she was unable to communicate, I turned to the Twenty-third Psalm. Conversation was no longer possible for Mom, and I don't know whether she still recognized me, but when she heard the familiar words "The Lord is my shepherd," a smile of recognition came to her and tension melted from face and hands.

And so it is with the imagery of this Psalm. It carries me still to a place of comfort, and to treasured memories of Mom and her faith.

Becky A Grover Ann Arbor, MI, USA
Moving Through Pain 62" x 14.5"

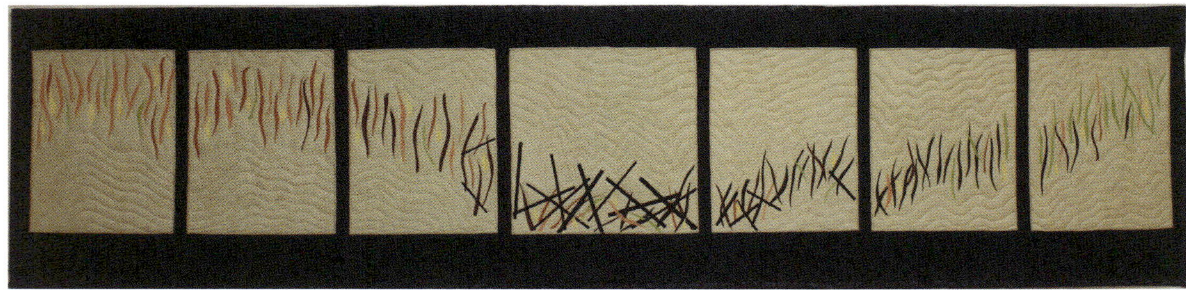

This piece is about the disruption that happens when pain comes into your life. The smooth flow of your routines becomes jagged; the colors of your life darken. As we move through the pain (of disease, death, loss, grief) we can again find happiness, but we are different. Our rhythm and colors have been changed by our experience.

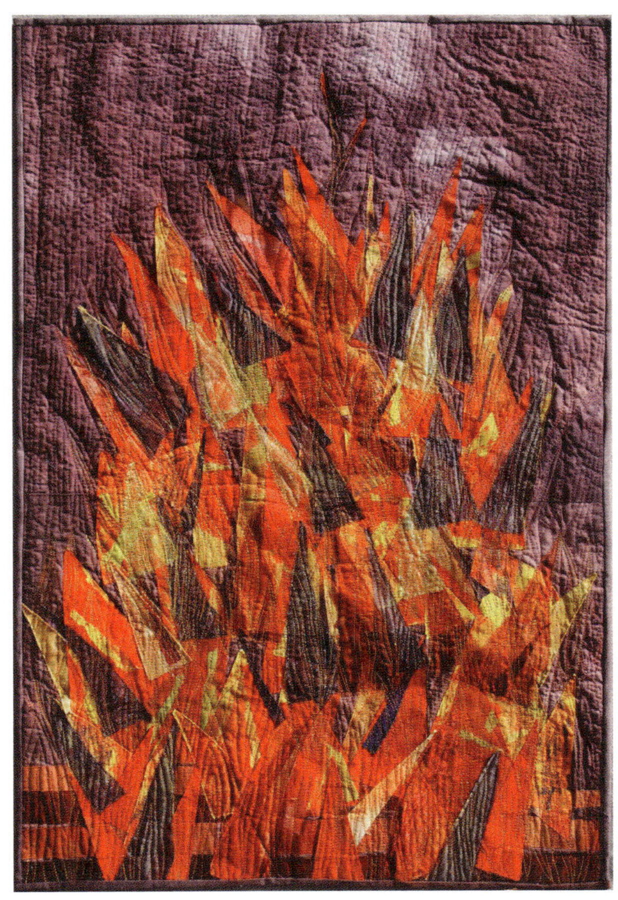

Barbara Eisenstein
Bethesda, MD, USA

Triangle Factory Fire Remembered
21" x 30"

The Triangle Shirtwaist Factory Fire of 1911 resulted in the loss of 146 lives, mostly young immigrant women. They were sweatshop workers, trapped in the upper floors of a New York building with locked doors. For me, this horrific event has particular significance as my grandmother a factory worker, witnessed the fire and watched many victims jump to their deaths. With this quilt, I commemorate her experience. She lived and worked to see a turning point in conditions for workers, with unionization and formation of commissions to regulate working conditions.

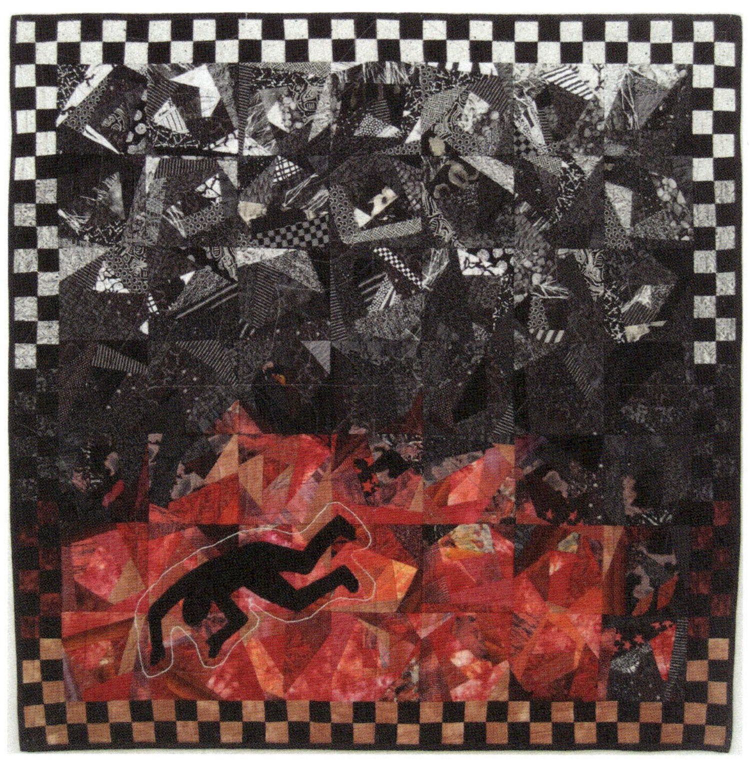

Helena Scheffer   Beaconsfield, Quebec, Canada
Catharsis 39.5" x 39.5"

Making this quilt helped me move past the negative emotions I felt after my husband was unjustly accused of corporate theft by the thief himself. I wrote the criminal's name with bleach on black fabric and sliced it up, including it in the quilt. He is the figure surrounded by crime scene tape, burning in the fires of hell, caught in his web of lies. I felt so much better after completing this piece!

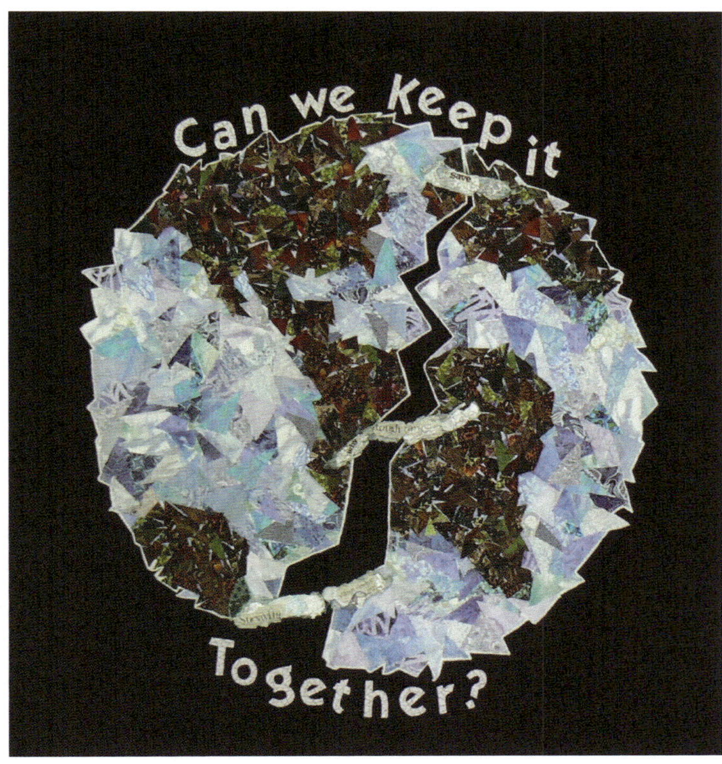

Wendy Butler Berns
Lake Mills, WI, USA

Can We Keep it Together?
42" x 43"

"None of us has it all together, but together we have it all." --- Author unknown

The earth is in such a fragile state, but it is my hope that everyone can work to hold it together. We need to save resources, maintain green spaces, conserve energy, reuse and recycle, protect the forests, wildlife, waterways and the air that we breathe. There are many generations ahead of us. For all to survive, the old gentle earth needs to be treated with tender loving care.

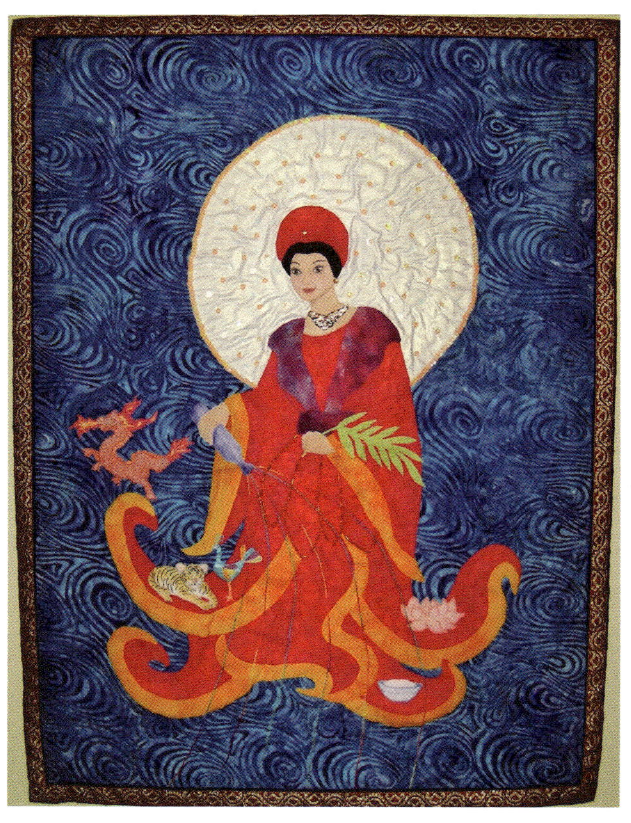

Juanita R Sauve
Ottawa, Ontario, Canada

Kuan Yin: Mother of Compassion
26" x 34"

Kuan Yin hears the cries of the world, loves all beings, and feels the plight of others as if it were her own. Here she holds a willow branch, sprinkles the nectar of life, pictured with rice bowl, lotus flower (pure heart), dragon (spirituality). Bird rests beside tiger.

I was inspired by a Vietnamese woman's story of a miraculous escape when pirates boarded a boat filled with refugees. Frightened, the refugees chanted Kuan Yin's name. Seeing a picture of Kuan Yin in the boat, the pirates left without harming anyone. Practicing compassion towards ourselves and others has the power to heal the world.

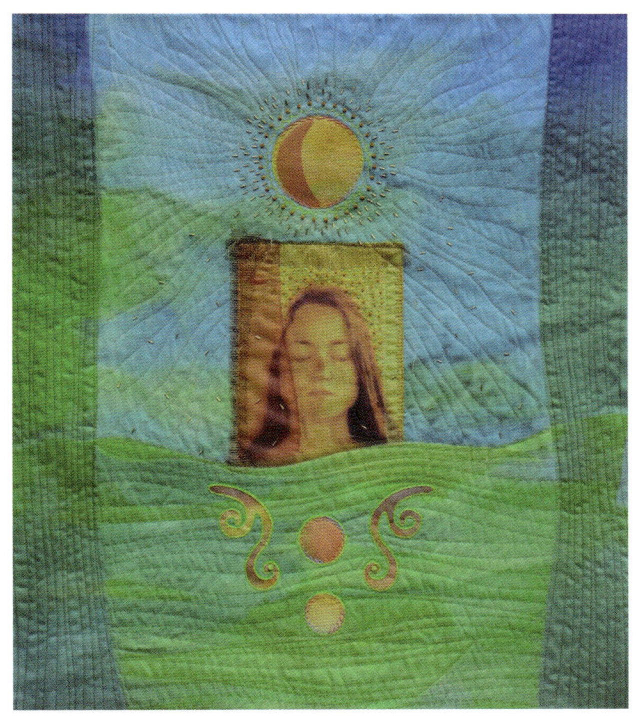

Sherrie L Spangler
Gig Harbor, WA, USA

Spring Meditation
28" x 31"

Winters in the Pacific Northwest are long, grey, drizzly, dark and (for me) depressing. When the darkness really gets to me, I close my eyes and meditate on the clear fresh light of spring. I imagine warm breezes and sunlight filling the days, bringing peace and new life and clearing away the winter darkness. The photo is one of my daughter, who is in the spring of her life. I added a warm cast to the picture and painted fabrics in spring greens, clear sky blues and golden orange. Shimmery beads and metallic threads reflect light.

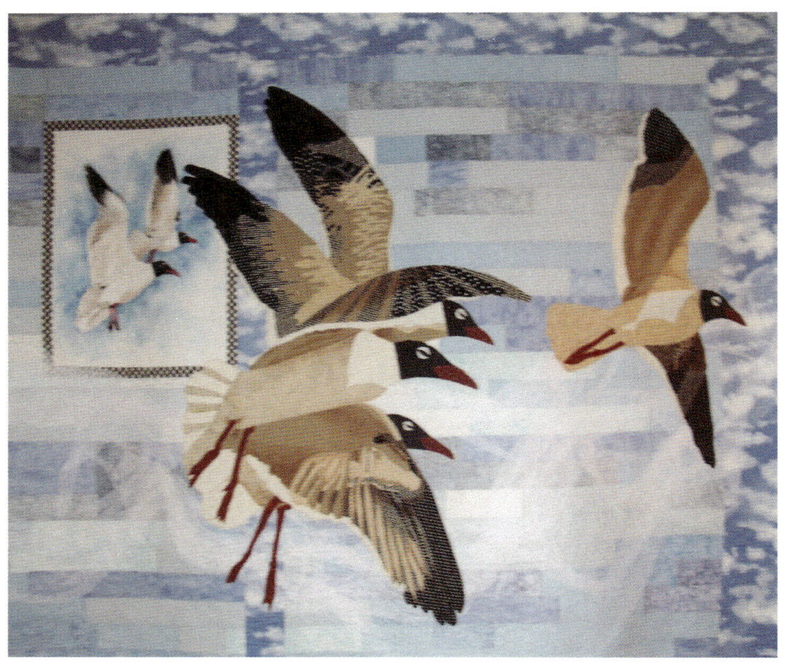

Dianne E Thomas Fairfax, VA, USA
From Papa's Window 58" x 47.5"

My father-in-law, Papa, participated in an atomic-bomb test at Eniwetok in 1945. Years later a tumor was removed from his spine; eventually walking became impossible and he was in constant pain. When he retired to the Florida Gulf coast, every day from his kitchen window he watched sunsets, dolphins, and sea birds. In his last years he became the father I never had, offering guidance and encouragement until his death in 2011.

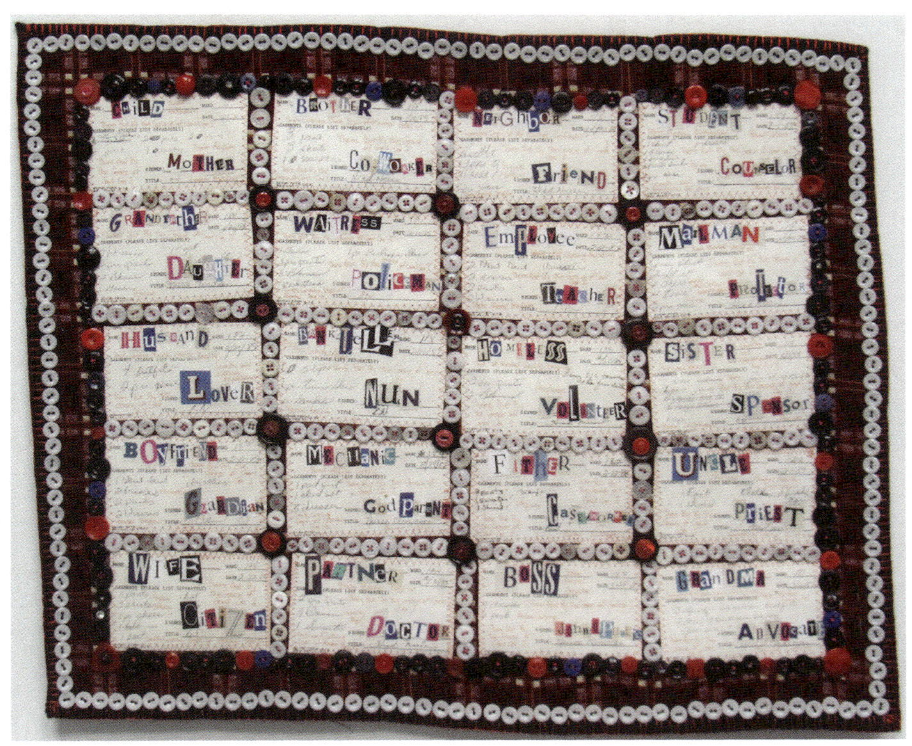

Susan Lenz Columbia, SC, USA
There But By the Grace of God 28" x 21"

The index cards and buttons were salvaged (with permission) from the now abandoned, historic South Carolina State Asylum's laundry and clothing department. Each was altered to hide real staff and patient names. The process of turning these cards into art was a spiritual journey, one recognizing the frailty of life and mental health. Creating a quilt was an act of comfort. Stitching the pieces together required a spiritual patience, love and an understanding of "There But By the Grace of God Go I."

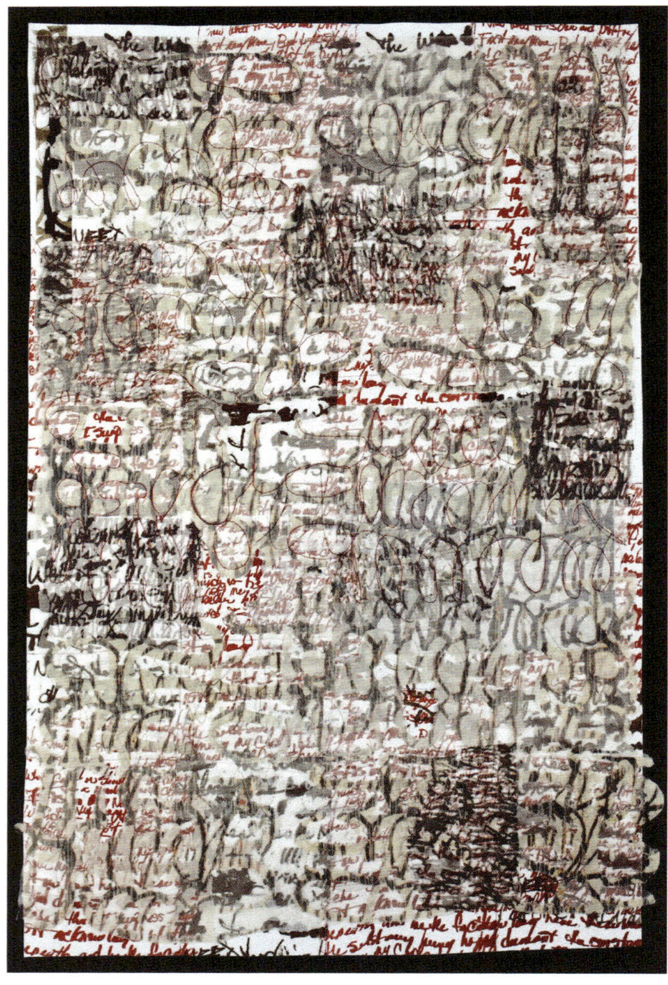

Denise Linet
Brunswick, ME, USA

Letters to Myself-
Page 3
26" x 39"

Having broken my wrist in the winter of 2011, I spent a lot of time writing in my journal about my recovery process and the meaning of mark making and its importance to my art making. I needed to record my journey back to healing. I needed to reflect on the marvelous organism that our body is, how it heals, the intricate functions of bone, muscle, tendon and nerves. My artwork has become the documentation of the role the mind/spirit plays in the healing process through journal writing, notes, poems and reflection.

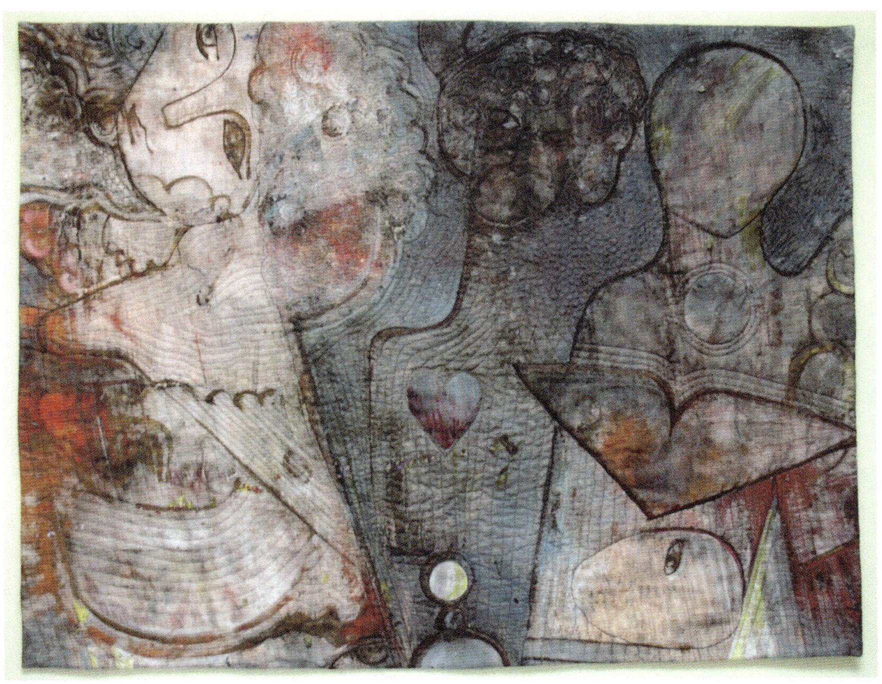

Karen S Musgrave Naperville, IL, USA
Glimpses of the Dark Angel 40" x 30"

Thomas Mann said, "Depression has its own angel, a guiding spirit, whose job it is to carry the soul away to remote places where it finds unique insights and enjoys a special vision." It took me more than thirty years to embrace his wisdom and truly understand. It made all the difference.

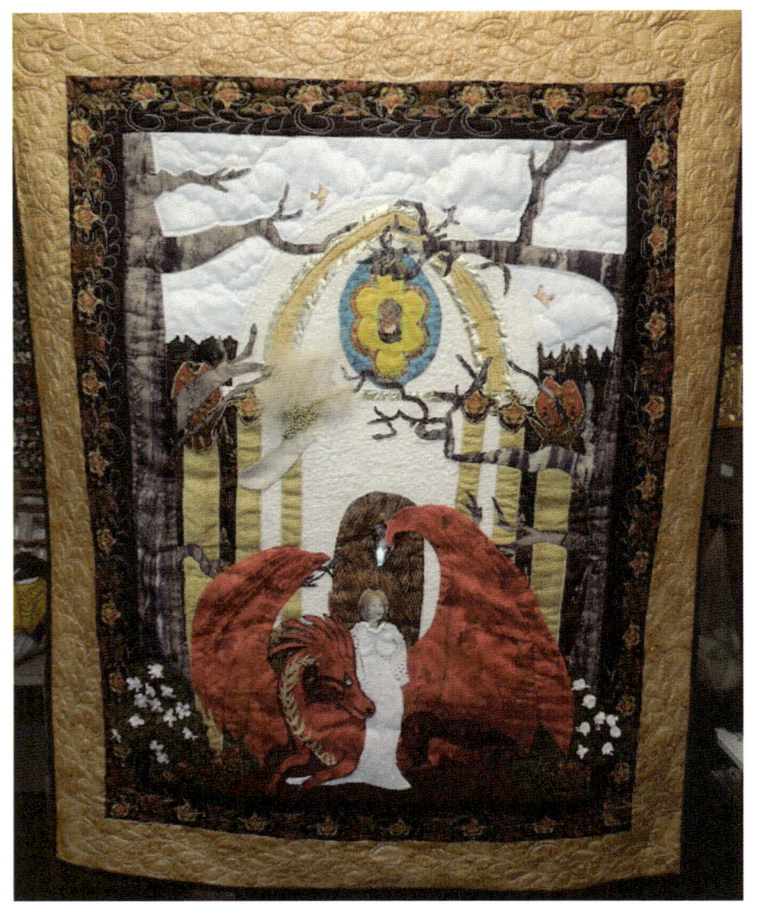

Watana Cantrell
Vernon, AL, USA

Lita Slaying her Dragon, Cancer
34” x 42”

I made this quilt in honor of our daughter, Lita, who has been fighting a Glioblastoma brain cancer for the past 3 years. The Dragon represents cancer, which she has tamed but not yet slain. The chapel behind is her place to pray, the doves in the sky give her peace, the flowers on each side are a love of hers, the feathered wing Guardian Angel above her has had her in his care since the beginning of the journey. She is still fighting this battle; but seems the Dragon is getting stronger, day by day. Lita has a beautiful spirit.

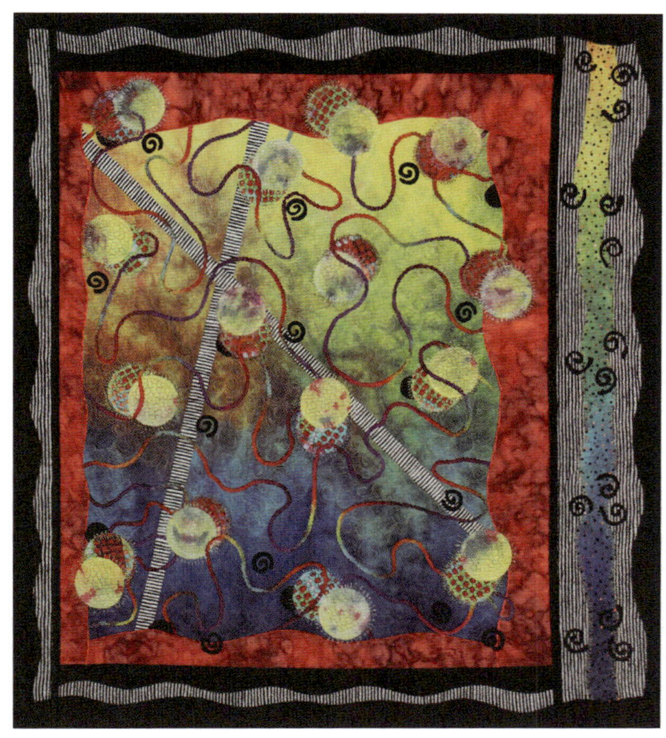

Judith Heyward
Hendersonville, NC, USA

Hidden Potential
42” x 47

“Hidden Potential” is a reminder that regular checkups for breast cancer are essential. We think everything is going along well and the sky is bright in our lives; however, beneath the surface lies the potential for cancer cells to be brewing. It is our responsibility to find them and have them removed so that there will be many, many more sunny days in our future.

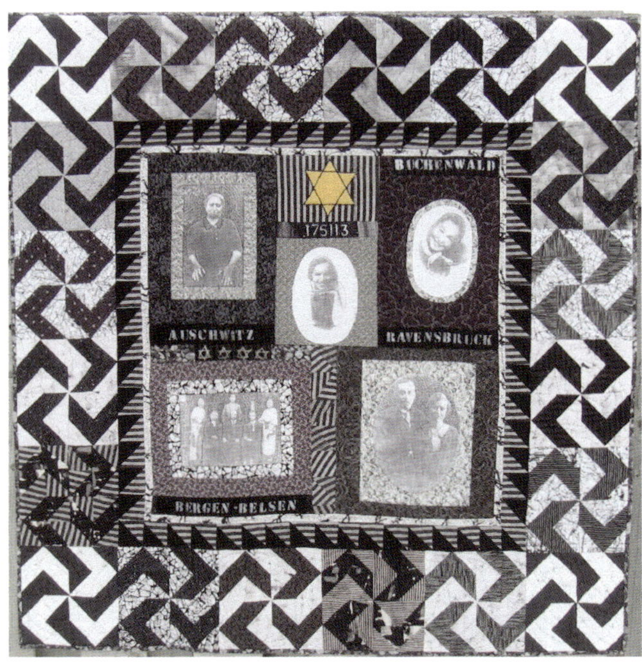

Helena Scheffer Beaconsfield , Quebec, Canada

Remembering My Family: A Holocaust Memorial Quilt

48" x 48"

This quilt is a personal tribute to my father's immediate family who perished in the concentration camps during World War II. It is also a memorial to the millions who lost their lives at Nazi hands. Working on this piece, especially quilting around the faces of the family members I was never able to know, was extremely difficult, yet made me feel closer to them.

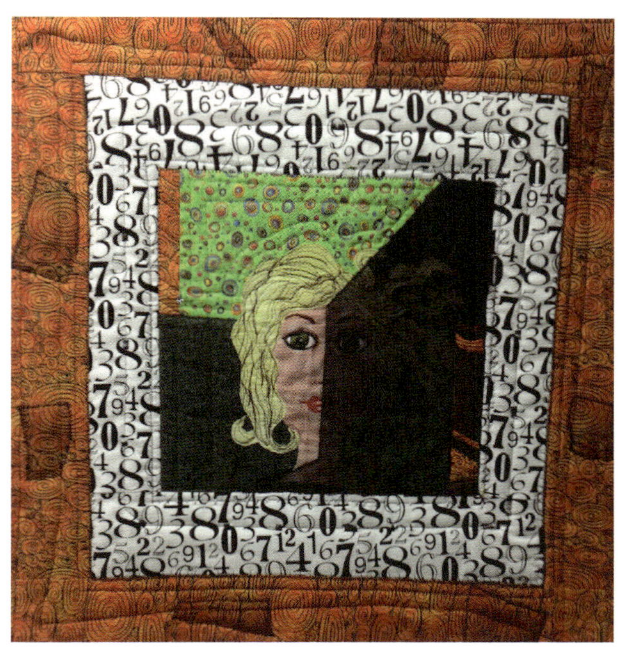

Kate Owens
Conroe, TX, USA

Understanding Mia
20.25" x 20.75"

Mood disorders affect our family. Some days are easier than others. I am learning to understand and cope with the disorder and how it affects not just the individual, but the entire family. It is not a death sentence, although it can be deadly if left untreated in some cases. Hence the darkness versus the happy side of her face. She can look fine on the outside, but be turbulent on the inside all at once. Good medicine and therapy have helped her find a sense of normalcy more often. The black netting on the border represents the cobwebs that clutter her thinking process when she's having an episode, and the other stitching represents healing wounds. I chose the numeric fabric to symbolize the "code" of our "computers" - our brain. Sometimes the code gets mixed up as reflected in the top row of upside down numbers. Various stitching represents heartbeats - life - and avoiding falling into the dark valley of suicide. The healing has begun and we celebrate that.

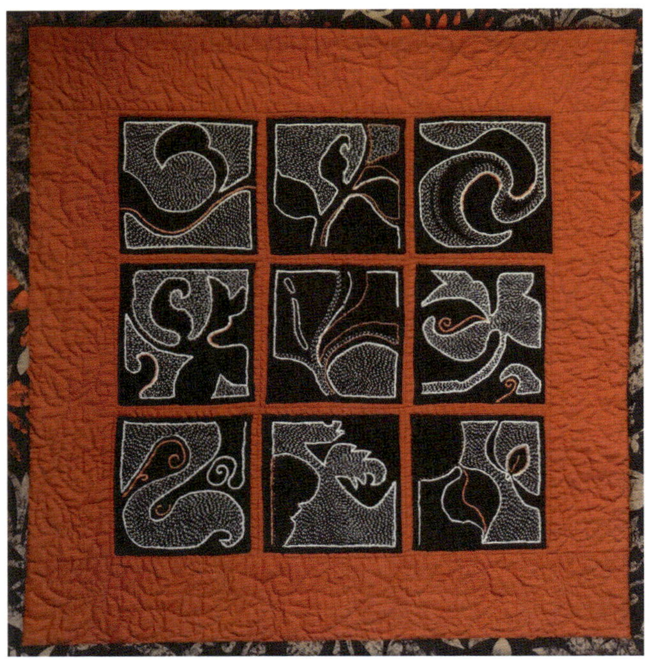

Kim Svoboda
New York, NY, USA

Kantha Leaves for FN
27" x 27"

For 11 years I accompanied my friend and mentor to dialysis - and stitched. I began this piece in the last year of FN's life. I knew that when I finished it, he would no longer be with us on earth. I carried these squares everywhere, from home to hospital rooms; rehab centers to vacation stays. Stitching gave me peace and allowed me to care for him in the ways he needed. I completed it on July 3, 2011, the day he passed away. He will be with us always.

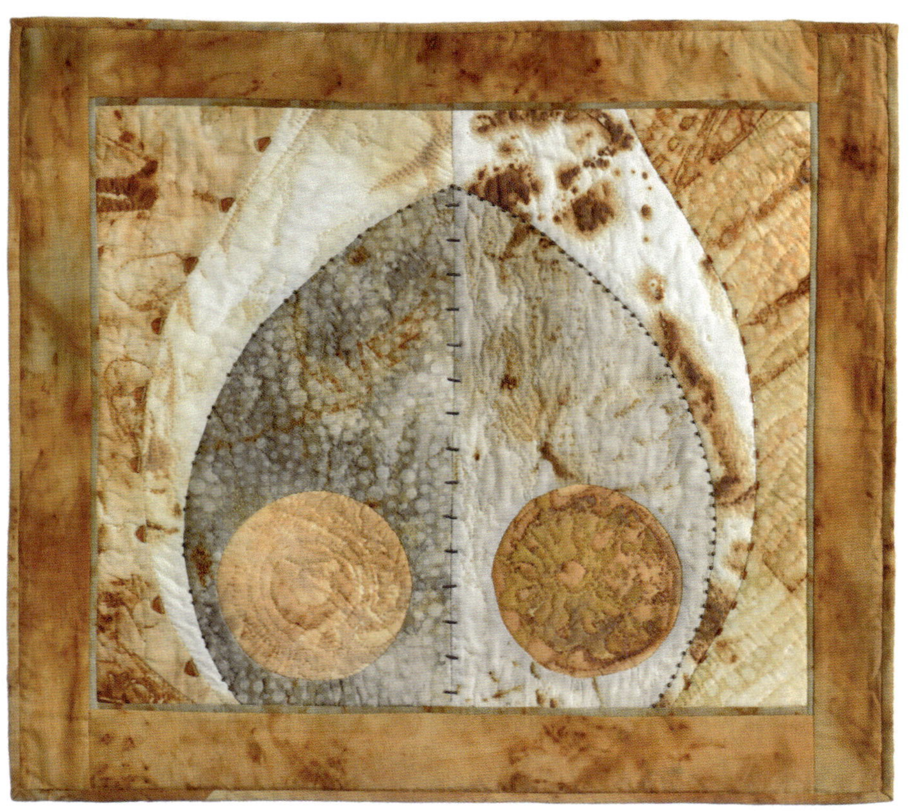

Candy A Flynn Middleton, WI, USA
Not All the Way Through 25" x 22"

"Not All The Way Through" reflects on the ways we grow, heal and become whole; seaming together our pieces, complete with scars and imperfections.

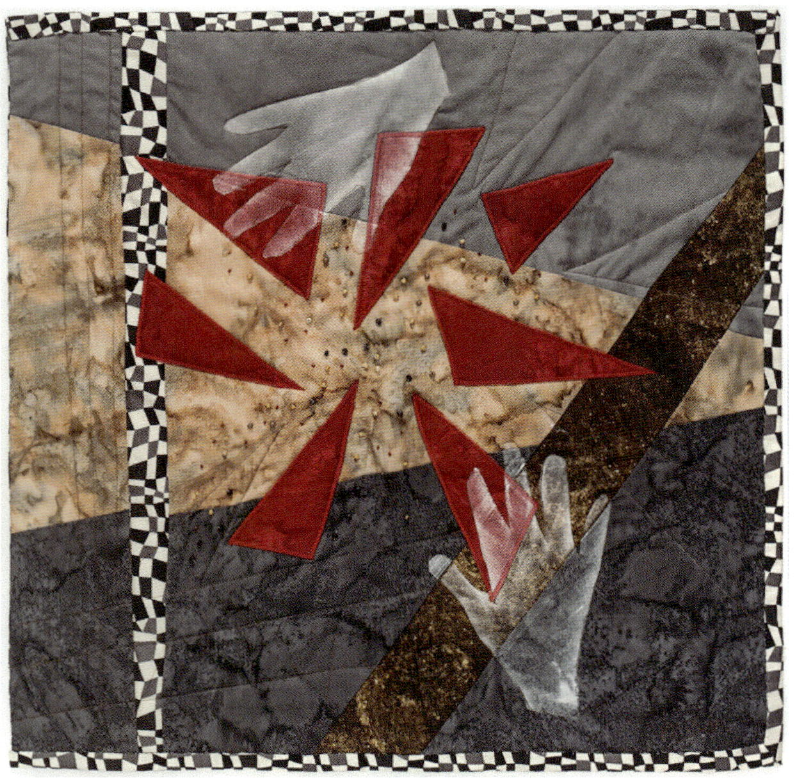

Kathy Mohan Melrose, MA, USA
Shattered 22" x 22"

When a young family member committed suicide, I turned to art to help process feelings of grief, disbelief, anger and sadness. Her life as well as many others is shattered. How can those left behind continue living? This piece is one step in a process toward healing and inner peace.

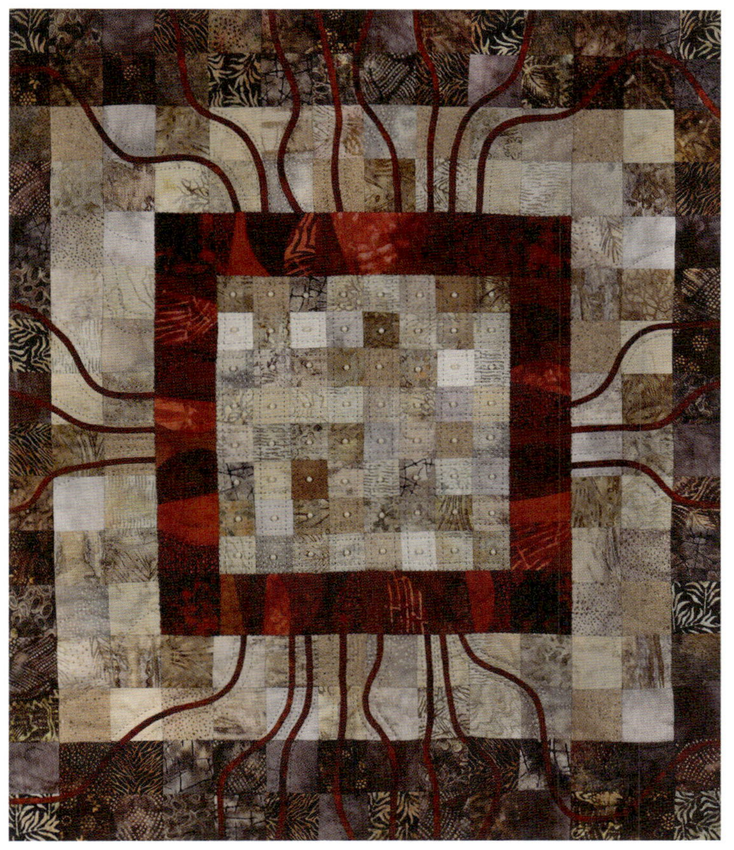

Anne Triguba
Westerville, Oho, USA

Suicide Dream
29" x 29"

After a long serious illness I thought about suicide constantly. One night I dreamed that I was creating a Broadway show called "Suicide". In my dream I made a quilt to be the motif for the show. When I woke I made a drawing, and then I created the actual quilt from my dream. Upon completion of the quilt the thoughts of suicide ceased.

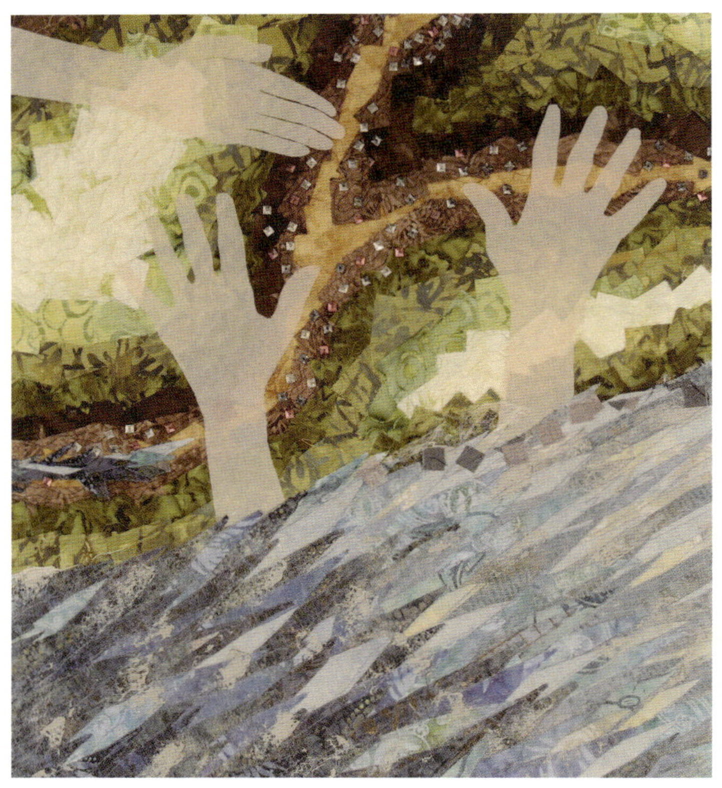

Meghan J Welch Arlington, VA, USA
Tsunami 23.75" x 25.75"

This quilt "Tsunami" was created in response to the Japan earthquake and tsunami in 2011, and was inspired by memories of providing aid after the 2005 tsunami in Indonesia. Vast tracts of land, homes, families, and livelihoods were swept away by nature. In the aftermath, diverse communities lent assistance to begin the rebuilding and healing process.

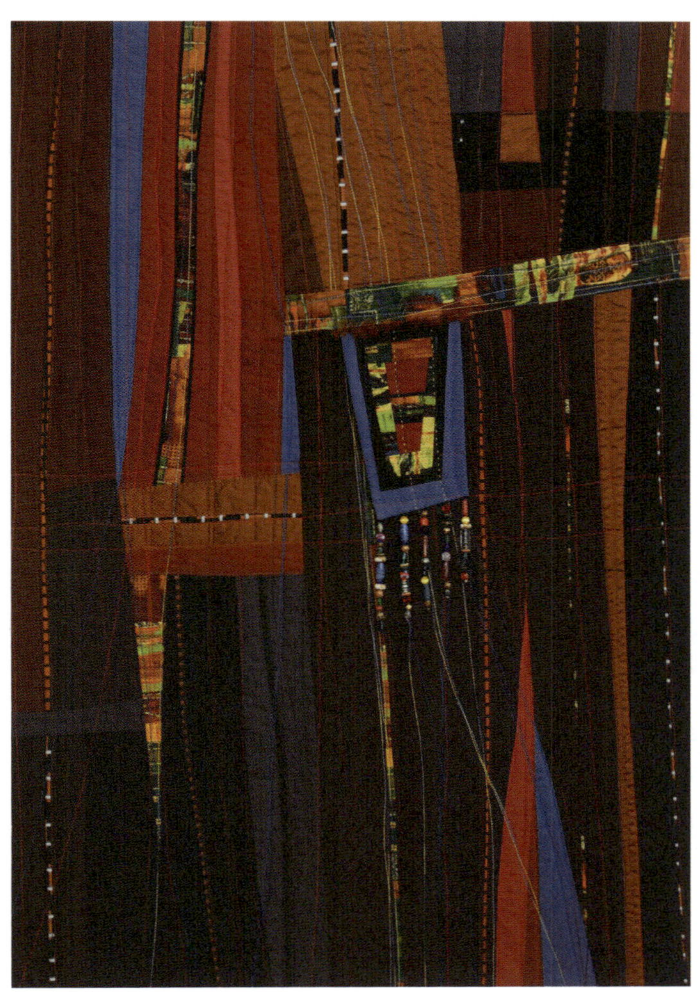

Cheryl Costley
Bonita Springs, FL, USA

Healing Pathway
29” x 41”

During the creation of this piece, I was praying for healing for my sister who was going through chemo for Stage IV ovarian cancer. In my mind the focal point became a protective amulet.

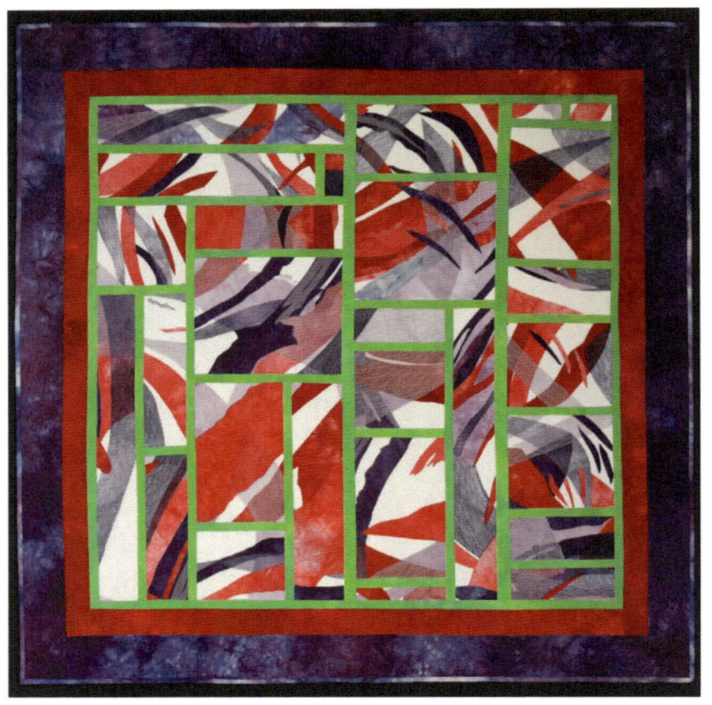

Jules Rushing
Lantana, TX, USA

Shattered Curves
40" x 39"

We all have moments when we are living comfortably, but when the unthinkable happens our comfort shatters. We struggle to put the pieces back together and are thankful for the guiding hands of God. Little did I know when creating Shattered Curves that God was creating through me and preparing me for my husbands' diagnosis of Mild Cognitive Impairment (Alzheimer's) at age 57. This quilt now represents my life. When the flow of life isn't working, it is time to step back and understand that God has a path for us that is sometimes uncomfortable.

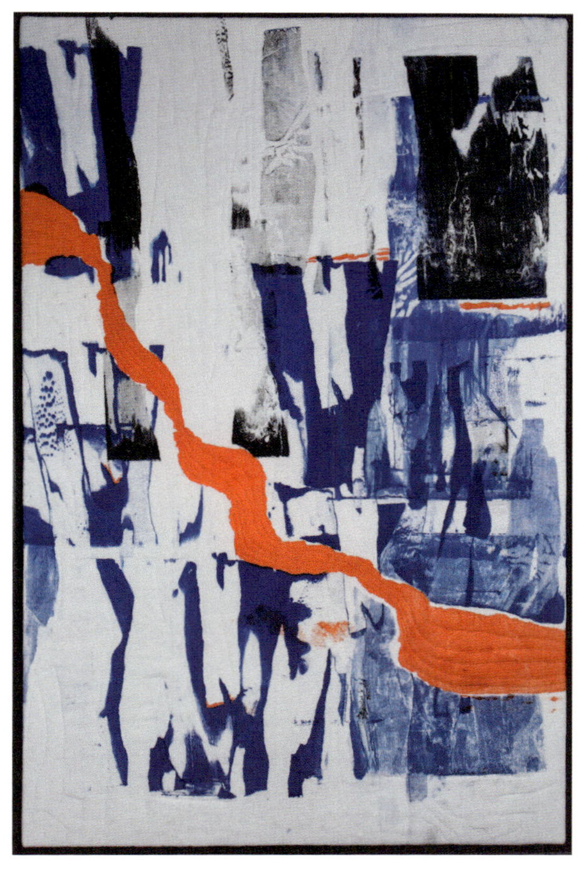

Sharon C Collins
Arnprior, Ontario, Canada

What Lies Beneath
24" x 36"

While I was silk screening for a piece inspired by lava and ice, I received a phone call that a dear friend had passed away. When I returned later to work on this piece it brought back all the emotions of that day. The pain and sadness of my loss was represented by the icy cold blues and hard blacks.This was contrasted with the warm orange of the lava,which symbolized my deep feelings and wonderful memories of our friendship. The stitching began the healing process and has come to represent our life bond to me.

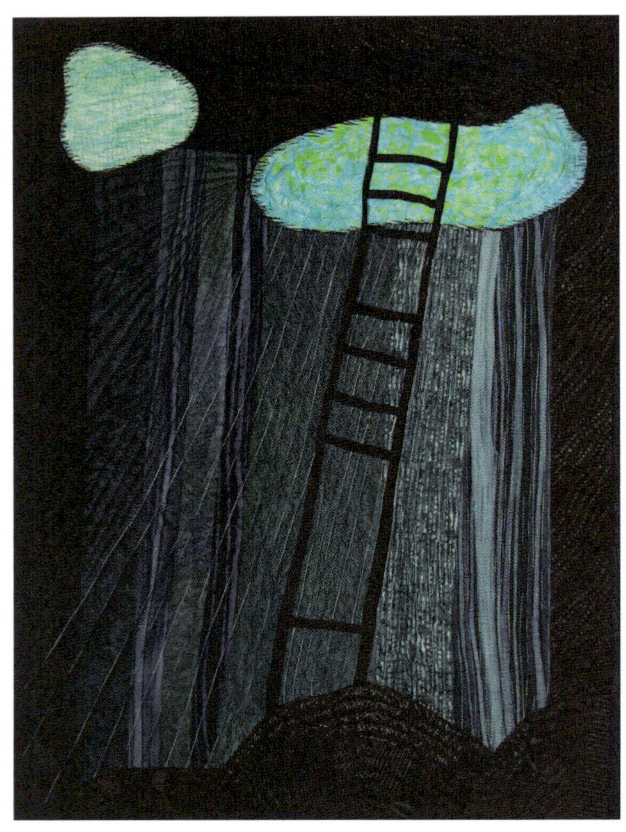

Nancy Feve
Bethesda, MD, USA

Stairway to Heaven
26" x 34"

This quilt is a memorial tribute to a cherished friend who died in a cave diving accident, and the only pictorial quilt I have ever attempted. It represents my long-fought acceptance of her leaving us behind and my hope that her spirit found its way to that ladder.

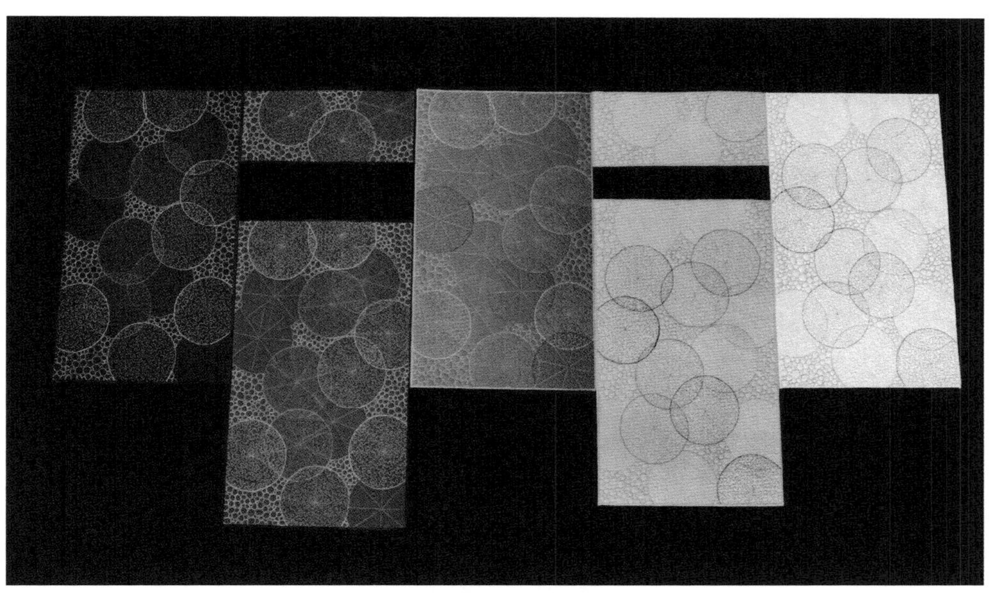

Marie Spadaro Centerville, MA, USA
Love and Loss 58.5" x 28.5"

After the vivid moment of a death or tragedy itself comes the long process of learning a new pattern for living. We go on with our lives, but the fact of that loss can descend like a fog, lifting only slowly, in stages, as we move on.

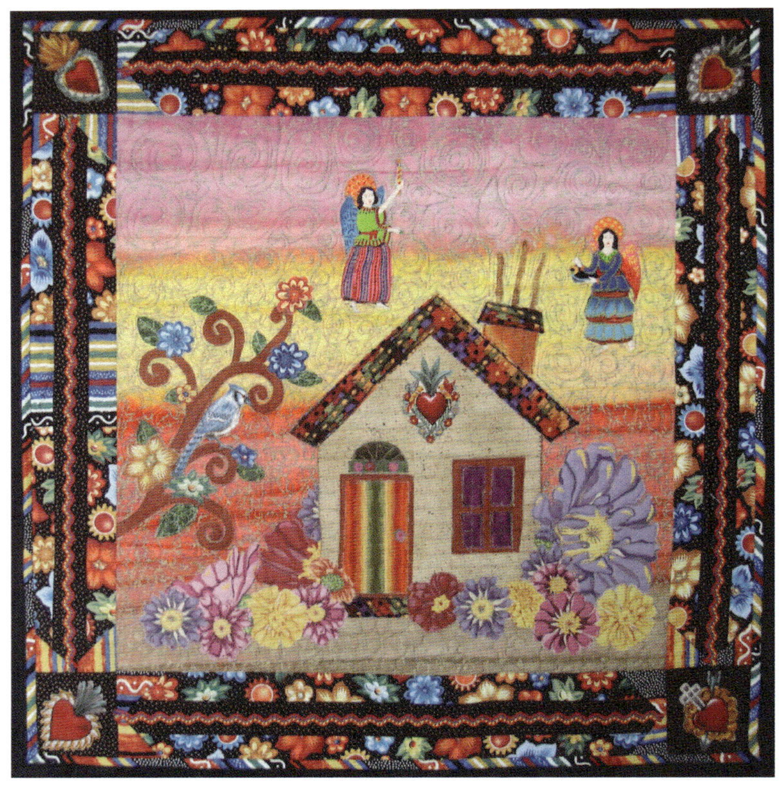

Elvia Dawson
Temecula, CA, USA

House of Memories
29" x 29"

Quilt was made to honor family and friends. Different symbols were used in their memory. Blue Jay - My father was everything to me and lost to suicide. Zinnias - My mother who taught me patience and resilience and I lost to surgery complications. Heart and Birds - My husband who was my soul mate, blessed me with two sons and lost his battle to kidney cancer. Angel with Key - My Nana. She was my rock, my teacher and lived to 99 years old. Angel with Candle - My best friend who was always there for me and I lost her to esophageal cancer.

Like the butterfly
I have the strength and the hope to believe
in time
I will emerge from my cocoon
Transformed

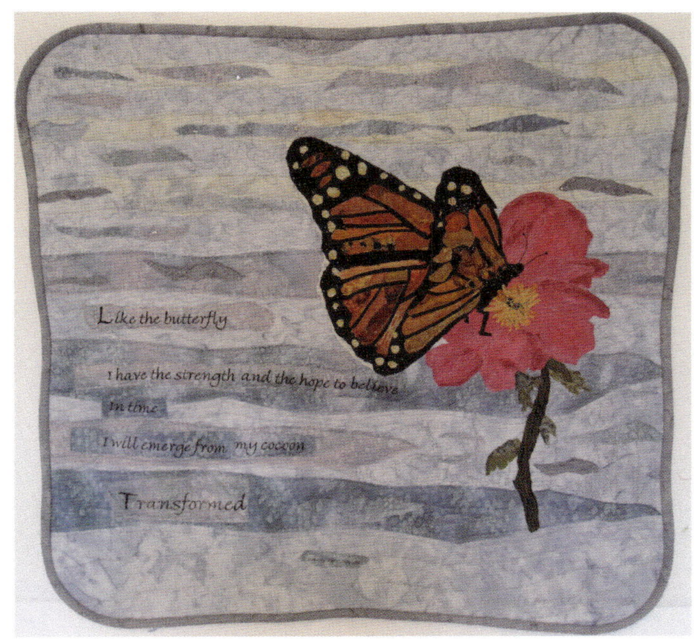

Dian B Epp
Spotsylvania, VA, USA

Transformed
25” x 24”

This quilt expresses my feelings a year after being diagnosed with Chronic Lymphocytic Leukemia (CLL). The diagnosis left me shocked, with questions, fears and a sense of loss. Since then I have embarked on a journey of discovery, making changes in my life that hopefully will lead to healing. Following a year of cocooning I feel it is time to venture out like a butterfly, transformed by what I have learned about myself. Hopefully, this insight will also allow me to live my life in a positive manner and accept whatever God's plan is for me.

SPIRITUALITY

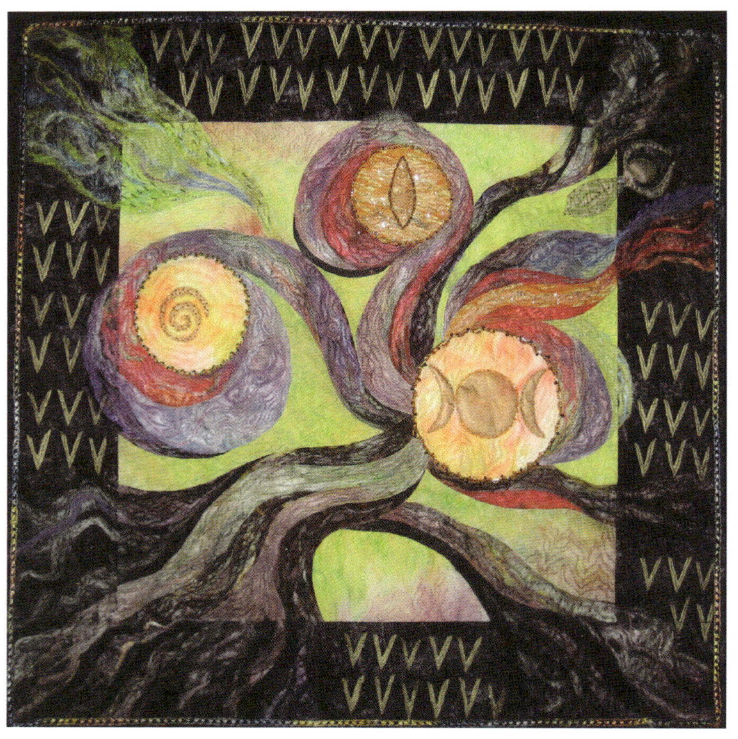

Karen S Riggins Versailles, KY, USA
The Feminine Embraces 30" x 30"

This quilt is a celebration of the "Sacred Feminine" that is in all of creation. In my spiritual journey I have come to realize that the spiritual feminine is ever present in our lives. She is nurturing and loving and all that is fertile and good. She is strong and is here represented as a strongly rooted tree that holds Love, Divine Wisdom and Creativity. She is us and we are her in all the beauty of creation and in all our daily lives.

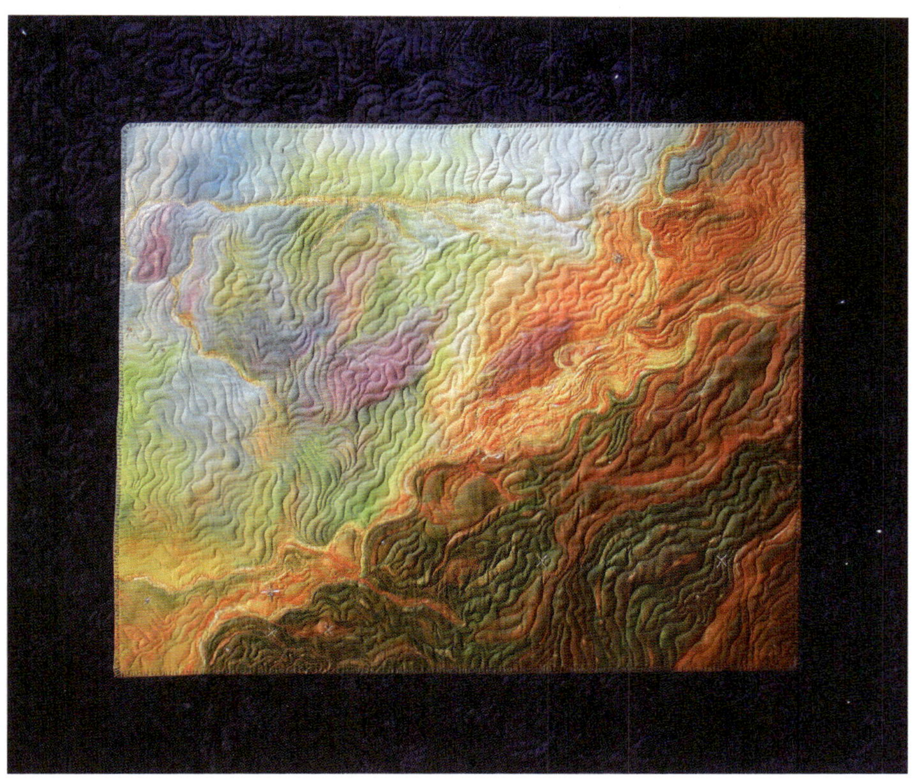

Sally G Wright Los Angeles, CA, USA
2009 - A Space Odyssey 38" x 31"

A NASA photograph from the Hubble Space Telescope - ("A Perfect Storm of Turbulent Gasses in the Omega/Swan Nebula") inspired me to create my version as a painted wholecloth quilt. I was astounded by the transcendent beauty of these images from another world we little understand. They can only serve to convince us of the hand of a higher power in its, and our own, creation.

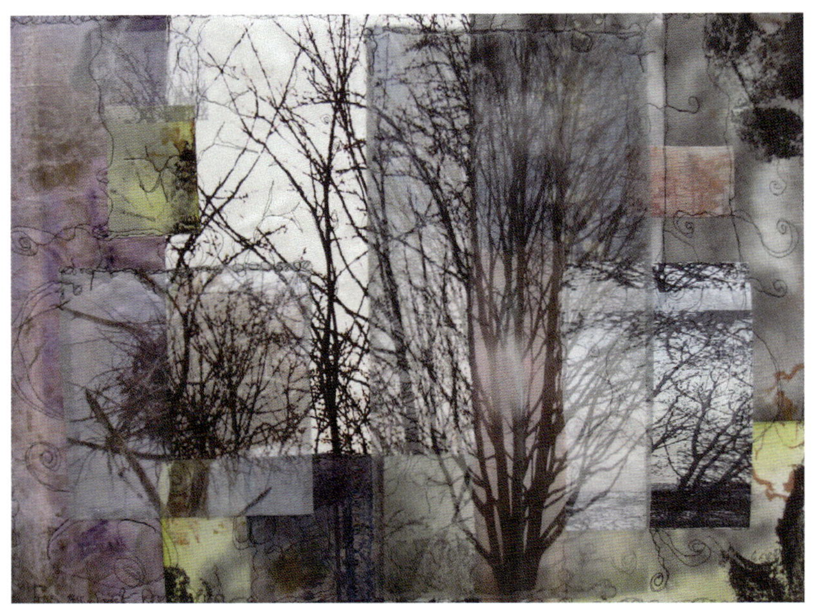

Wen Redmond Strafford, NH, USA
Trees Seen, Forest Remembered 33" x 24"

When I feel spaced out, tired, I go for walks.
Walks in among the trees reconnect me with spirit,
Change my perspective, remind me what's important.
To remember the forest

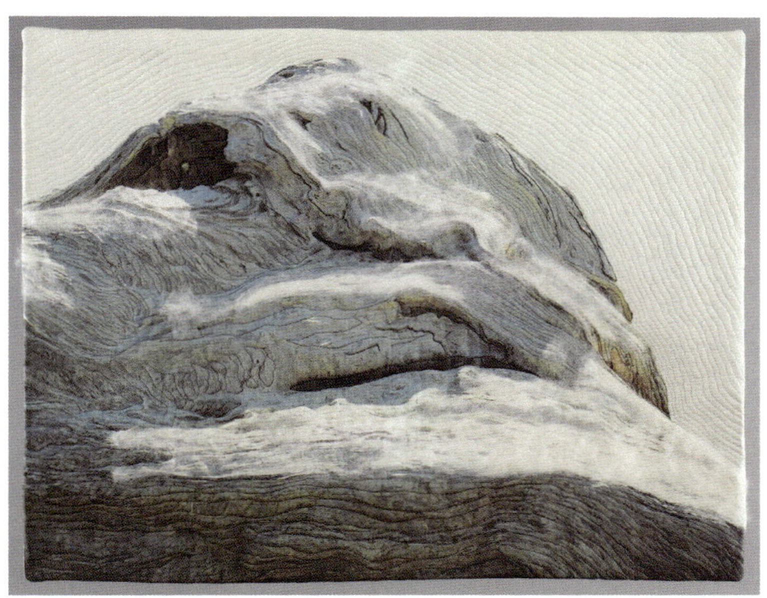

Judy Warner Victor, NY, USA
Spirit 29.5" x 22"

This piece speaks to me of spirituality - rising from a base of groundedness into the light and higher meaning. Our path may be complex, fraught with temptation and darker moments, but if we persevere, we will reach the summit.

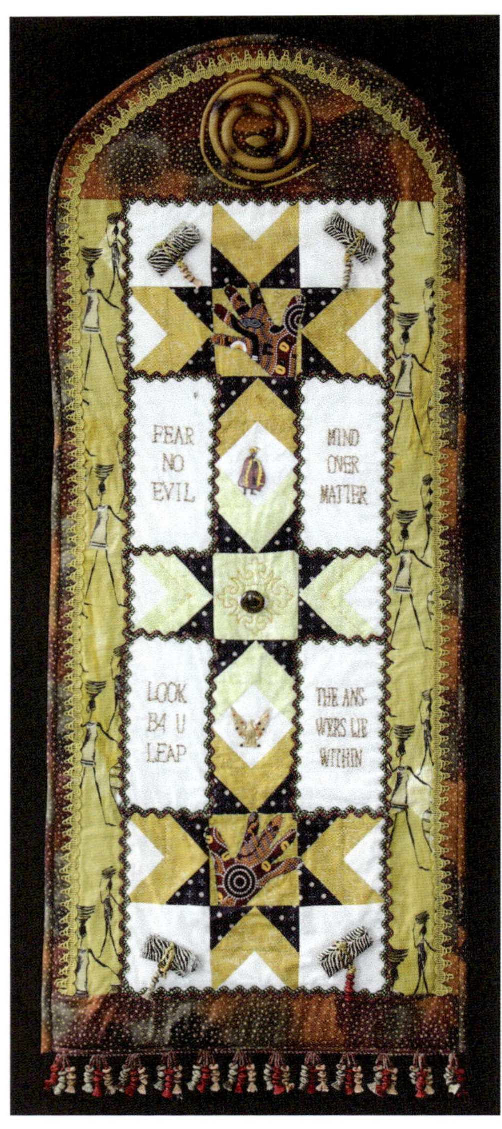

Meredith E Armstrong
Danville, PA, USA

Talisman
19.5" x 47.5"

Reading SACRED ARTS OF HAITIAN VODOU (Consentino) started me thinking about my own spiritual beliefs and symbols. I was raised by a Presbytarian and a Christian Scientist who gave me a sense of caution and taught me to think for myself. These influences are represented by the words on the piece, some visible, others invisible, in the scrolls: fear no evil, mind over matter, look before you leap, and the answers lie within. I incorporated symbols from my own history and other universal ones. All of these come together in "TALISMAN" creating a representation of my beliefs at this time.

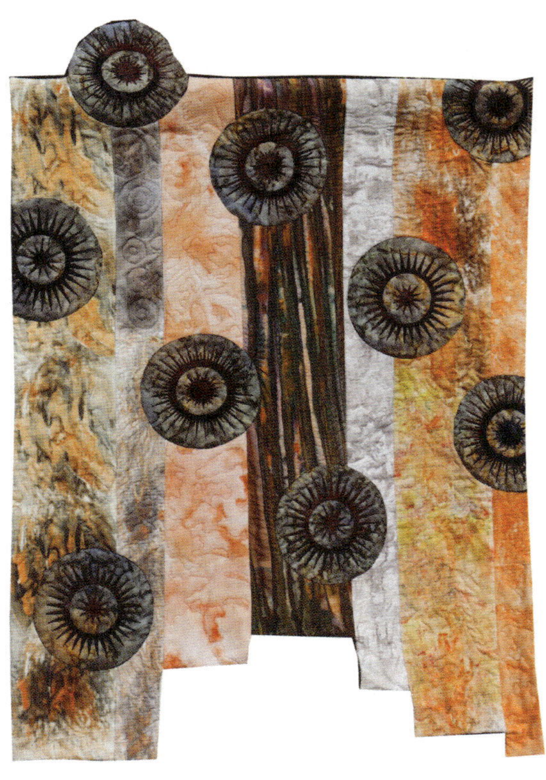

Sonia M Callahan
Piedmont, CA, USA

Gifts Of The Holy Spirit
33.5" x 47.5"

This quilt is meant to stimulate thought on the gifts we receive from the Holy Spirit. Although not always credited as coming from the Spirit,we receive these capacities and qualities in varying amounts as we travel on our spiritual jouneys. The nine circles represent gifts of the Holy Spirit: love, joy, peace, patience, generosity,faithfulness, gentleness, kindness, and self control. The circles are purposely not named as each person identifies a gift he/ she uses to bear fruit. These gifts enrich our lives and take on special meaning when shared in a society which does not always place these gifts in high esteem. The source of inspiration for this quilt comes from Ephesians 5:22 and Colossians 3:12-18.

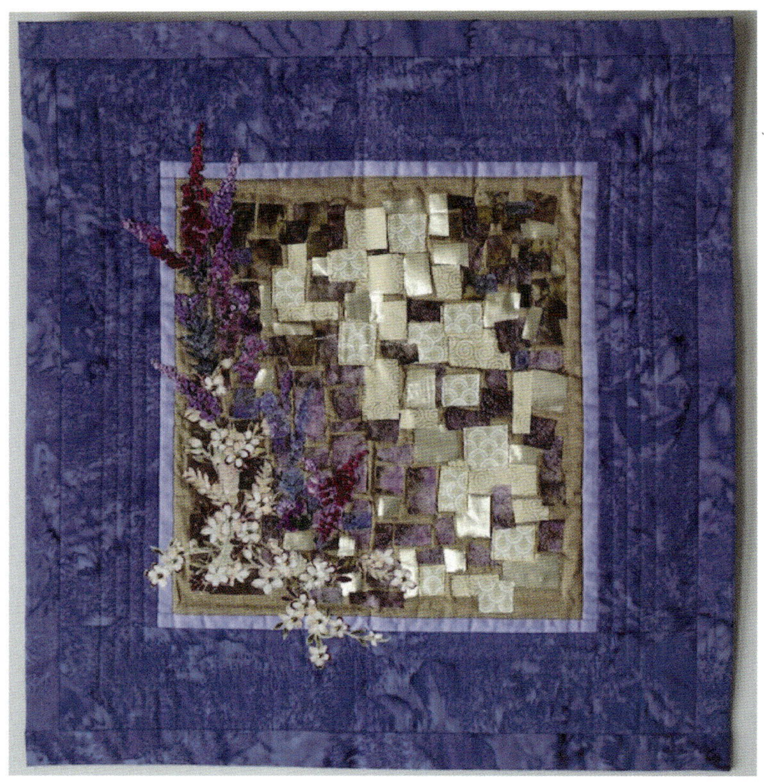

Ellie M Flaherty
Falls Church, VA, USA

A Little Grace For The Garden of My Soul
22" x 23"

What is this thing we call "grace"? One definition: "unmerited divine assistance given humans for their regeneration or sanctification." I like that, especially the word "unmerited". No cosmic score-keeping, no strings attached, just something for the soul, a spiritual boost if you will.

Here I picture my soul as a garden that needs something–not quite sure what–more courage? generosity? patience? –restored by an infusion of light and love. The grace that helps me do what needs to be done. What an amazing gift.

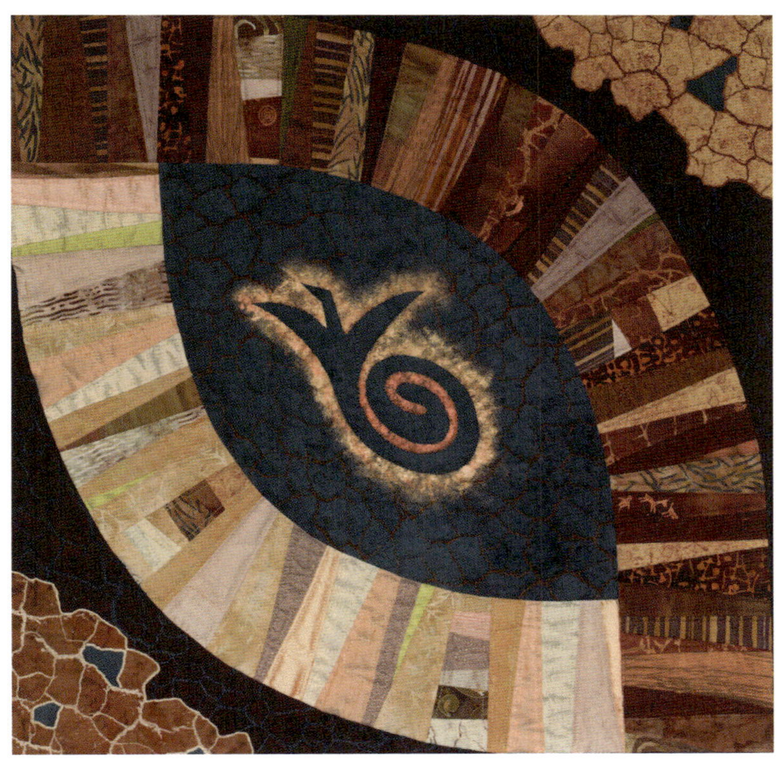

Sharon Rowley Seattle, WA, USA
Sun Eye 21" x 21"

This piece was inspired by a visit to the sacred place "Sun Eye" in Monument Valley Navajo Tribal Park. We were told that at celebrations the people would dance for 3 days and 3 nights. My original motif of the spiral crane, my spirit talisman of energy and health, is dancing in the hole in the rock formation which frames the deep blue sky of the Southwest Utah. The "red rock" is made up of layers of many shades of reds.

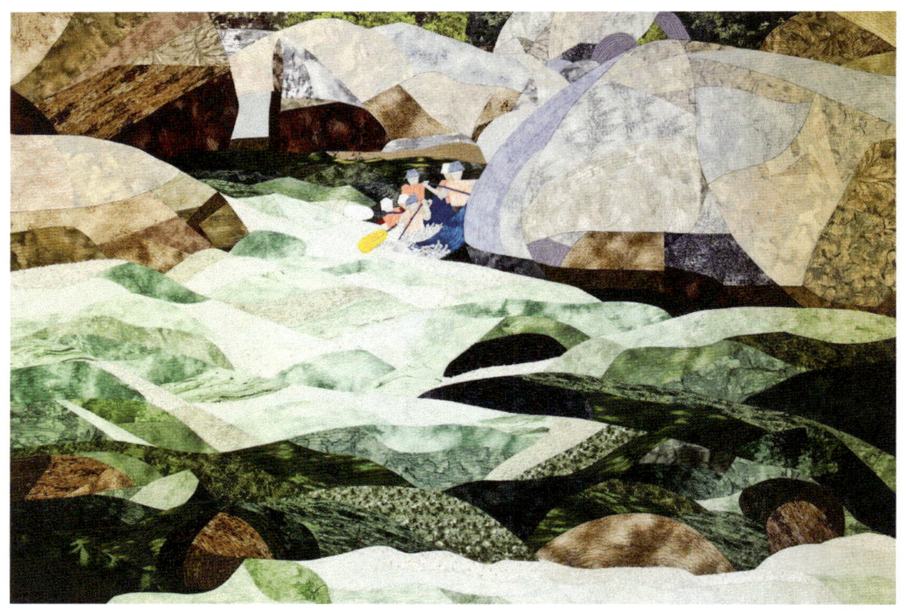

Suzanne Kistler Visalia, CA, USA
Through the Waters 70" x 47"

This quilt illustrates a terrifying journey through white water rapids, during which I fell out twice in the first five minutes. For the subsequent 2 hours, I was in a state of constant prayer, as I knew I was going to die that day. To say I felt close to God is an understatement.

The title comes from Isaiah 43:2 "When you pass through the waters, I will be with you." Thank God, He was.

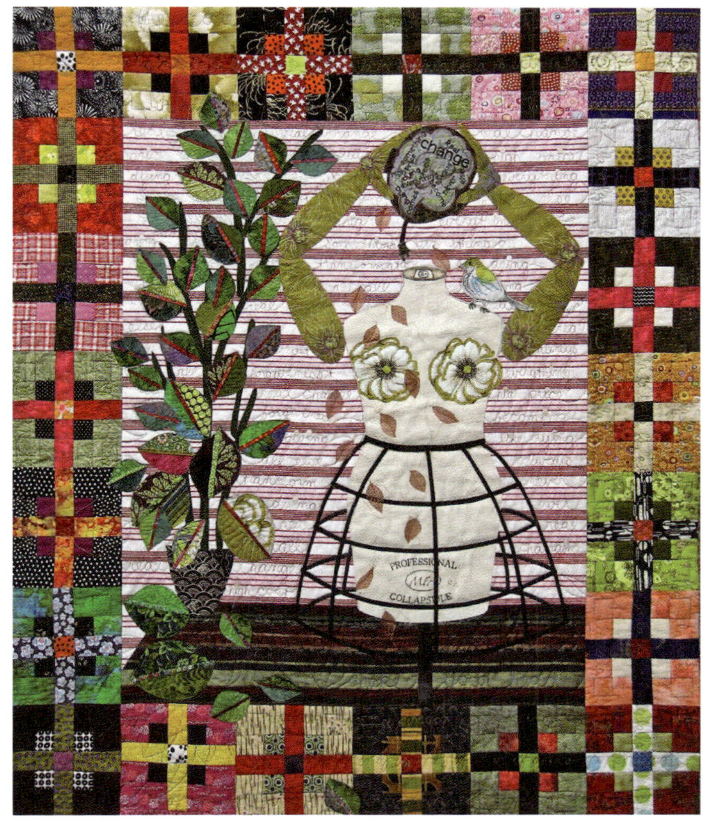

Karen Cunagin
Fallbrook, CA, USA

Change Your Mind
55” x 63”

CHANGE YOUR MIND. The natural world is ever giving itself up for the next cycle, as when fallen leaves become fresh soil. Contemporary knowledge and culture change before the sun sets. But Real (personal) Change never comes easily. Transformation, slow and painful in process, may feel like dying. You may have to take off your head and shake it.

I'm glad to be a woman and I like depicting the female form in regard to both physical and spiritual work. The mannequin's label, "Professional/ Collapsible," names our dueling strength and fragility. The caged skirt seems finite, unyielding; the bird suggests freedom and mercy.

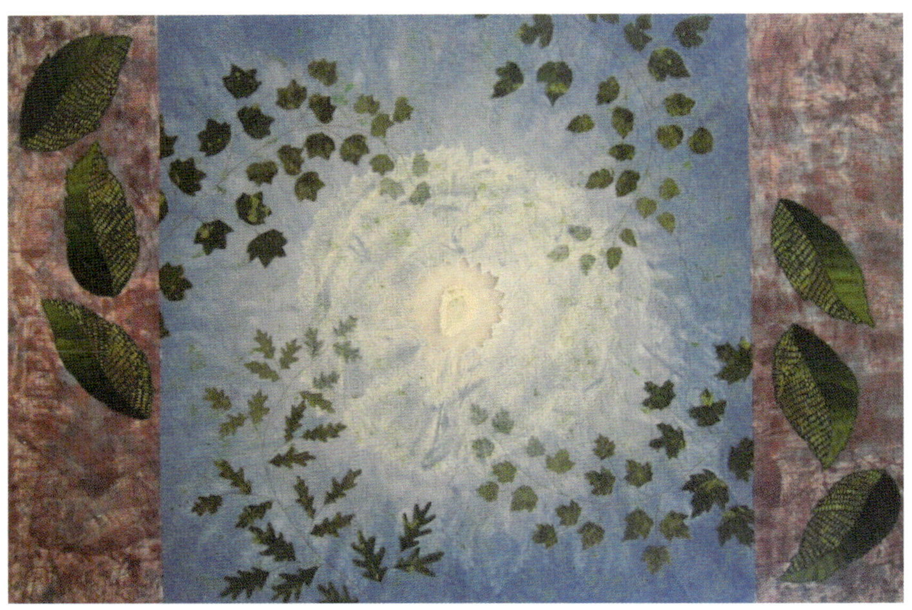

Eileen Doughty Vienna, VA, USA
Niggle's Leaf 64" x 43"

This was inspired by a short story, "Leaf by Niggle", by J.R.R. Tolkien, about humility, compassion and sacrifice, the pursuit of perfection and its just reward.

My fabric leaves strive towards the True Leaf, suspended within the quilt but not a part of it. The layers of the quilt drop away toward the center - exposing painted batting, and white netting.

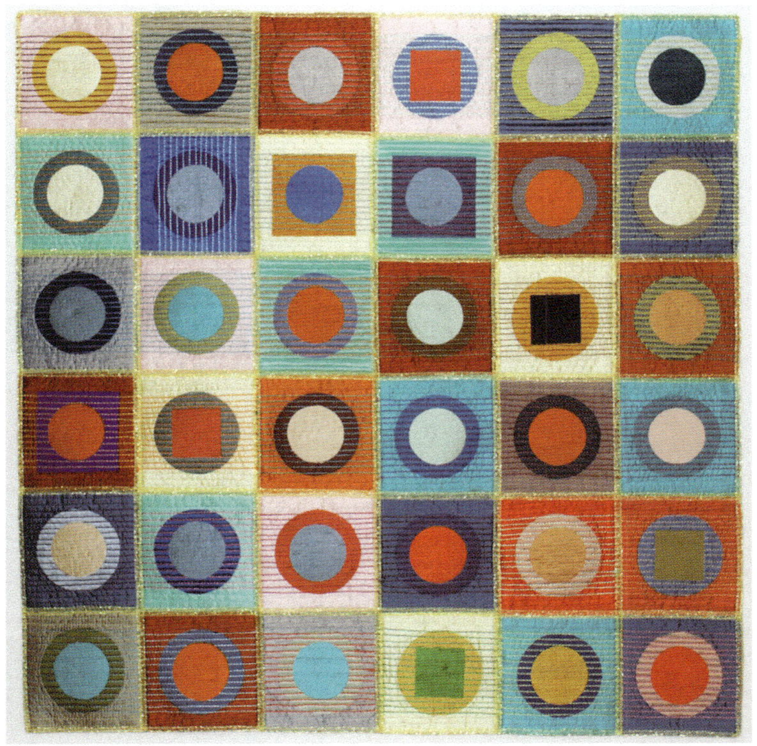

Susan Leonard Wynnewood, PA, USA
Silken Masks 25" x 25"

Our lives are less beautiful and orderly than we planned. Lurking behind--oft before--our lovely silken masks prowl demons that would control us. In other words, we would be those perfect round circles with strong connections to others were it not for those interfering shapes or voices that coach us to disconnect, to stay apart, to isolate in misery.

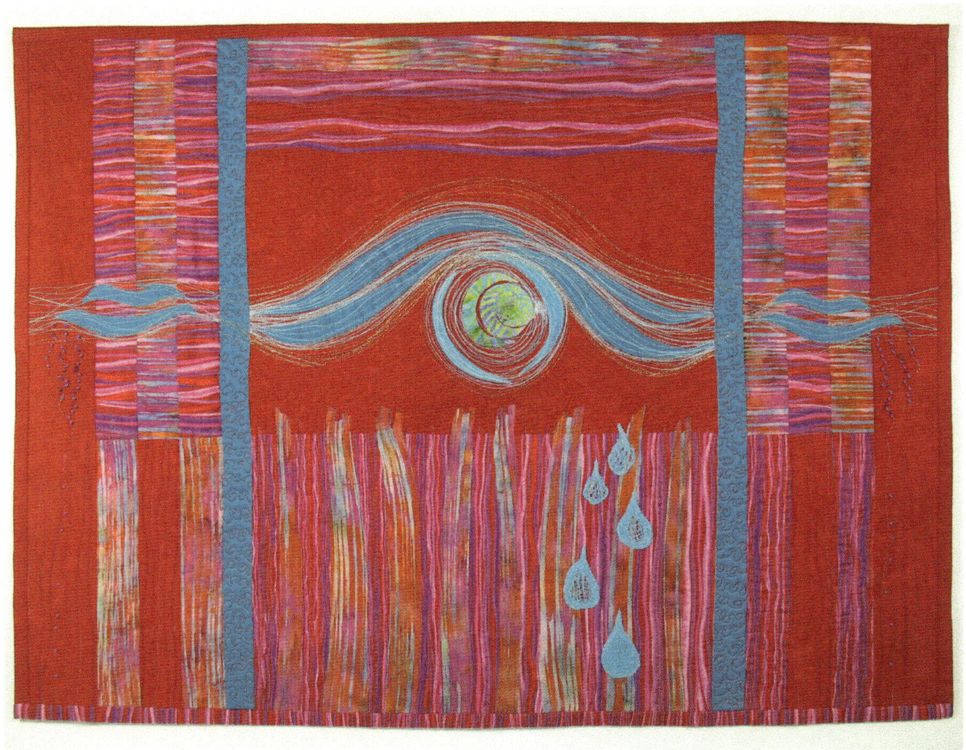

Linda A Miller Culver City, CA, USA
Heart's Vision 32.5" x 24"

There is an aspiration practice in the Buddhist tradition that asks: "May I be free from suffering. May you be free from suffering. May we be free from suffering." The intention is to contact genuine compassion. Connecting to the heart, in pain or joy, allows us to see the world more clearly.

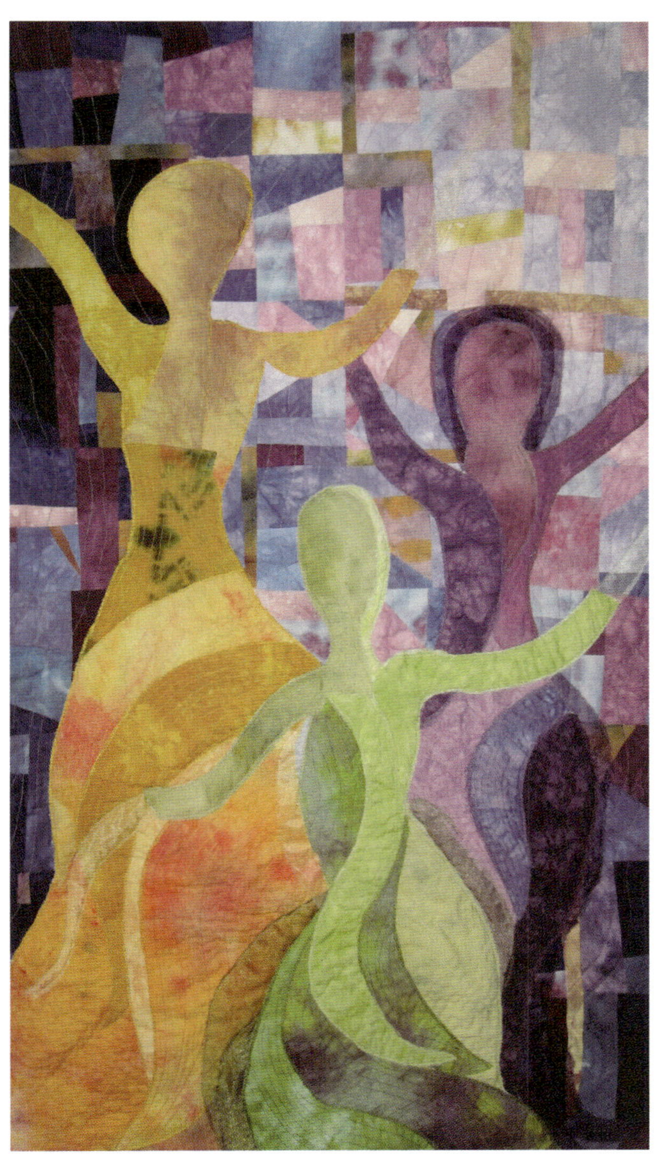

Nina-Marie Sayre
Albion, PA, USA

John 4:24
26.5" x 45"

"God is spirit, and his worshipers must worship in spirit and in truth." For without God, where would I be? He has had a hand in my life from the beginning, guiding me through the highs and lows of this world. I will praise Him with my last breath for without Him I am lost. This quilt was inspired by the praise and worship that resonates from my soul to the Heavenly Father.

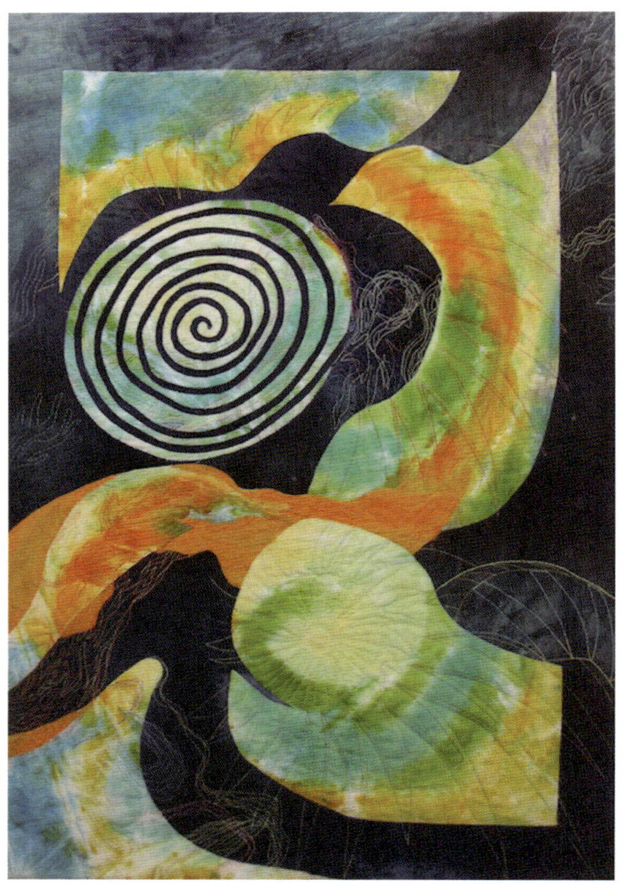

Christine B Smith
The Sea Ranch, CA, USA

Dualism Deconstructed
28" x 40"

This quilt is about integration. I quilted two dye-painted wholecloth quilts separately: representing my homes in suburbia and on the seacoast, one with tangled swirls, the other with a nautilus. Noticing anger and attachment, I cut each quilt into pieces and created a background/border integral to the design. A headless woman appeared, unable to speak, suggesting uncommunicated feelings. Intuitively I'd placed a spiral in the heart space. Spirit revealed that this symbolized my going in circles because of domestic conflicts. As the piece evolved, Spirit led me away from either/or thinking about my life, feelings, and perceptions of the Divine.

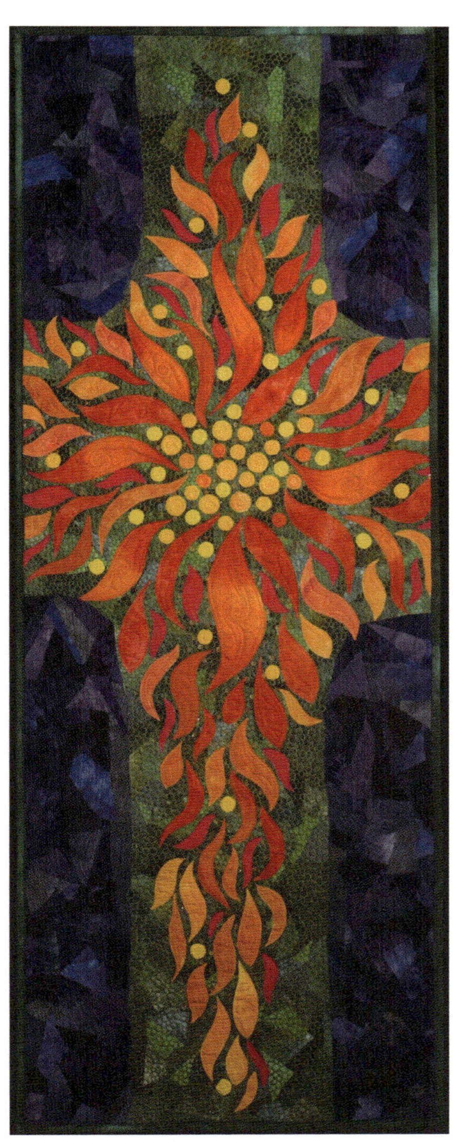

Larkin J Van Horn
Freeland, WA, USA

Pentecost
22.5" x 58"

The feast of Pentecost is one of a number of stories and commemorations that celebrate the bringing of light into a world waiting in darkness. Others are the Christmas star, the return of the sun following the winter solstice, the Genesis stories, and a myriad of creation myths. In this case, the light comes as tongues of fire to people standing at a crossroads of history and belief.

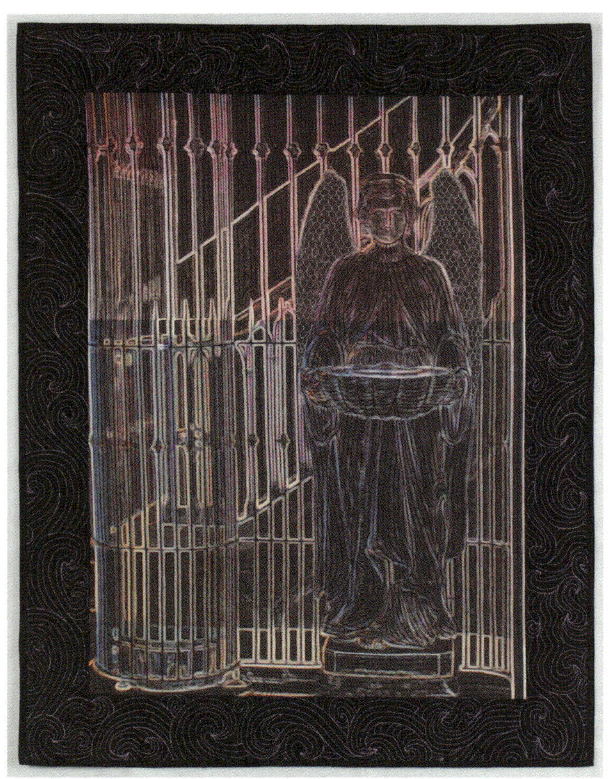

Virginia S Greaves Roswell, GA, USA
The Bowl Judgments 25.5" x 32.5"

In the deep recesses of the church, the statue of an angel glows. It is through her simple handling of the bowl that we are both asked to give of ourselves as well as reminded of the bowl judgments that will one day spill onto the earth in judgment of those that are greedy with their gifts.

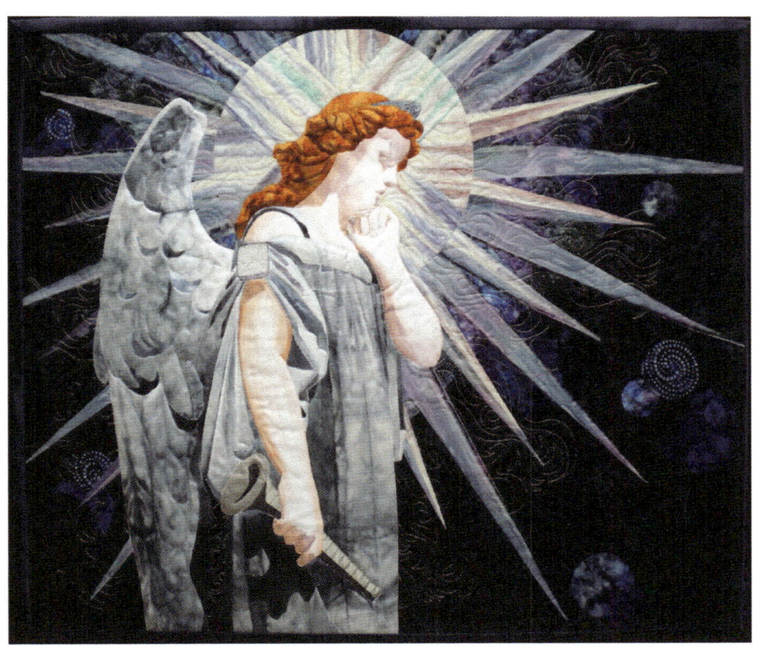

Melissa Sobotka Richardson, TX, USA
Archangel Haniel 43" x 36"

While visiting the cemetery after my father's death, I saw a monument of this angel. I found her to be so serene and peaceful. A photograph turned into a quilt and the statue came to life.

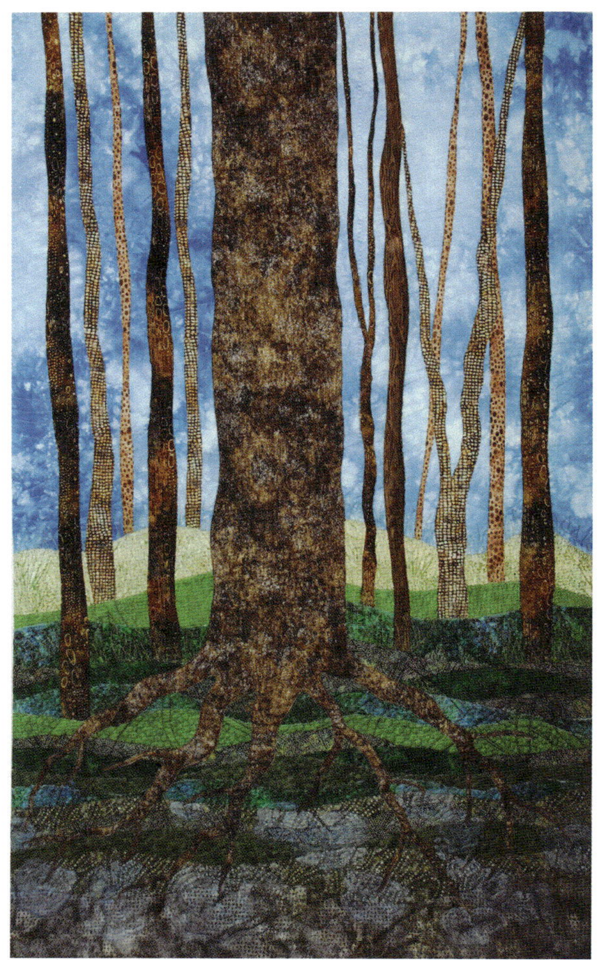

Karen A Brown
Westminster, MD, USA

Rootedness
35" x 55"

Trees are amazing creations, starting from a tiny seed, being nourished by water, sun and earth, reaching high toward the sky, and pushing below the surface. Roots develop and reach deep through dirt and rocks to provide grounding and seek out the nutrients needed to grow. We humans, too, are amazing. Our roots lead us deep into the past, connecting us to all who have been, all who have helped shape us and all who point us toward the future. Whether smooth or garbled, our roots have helped us grow tall and point to the sky.

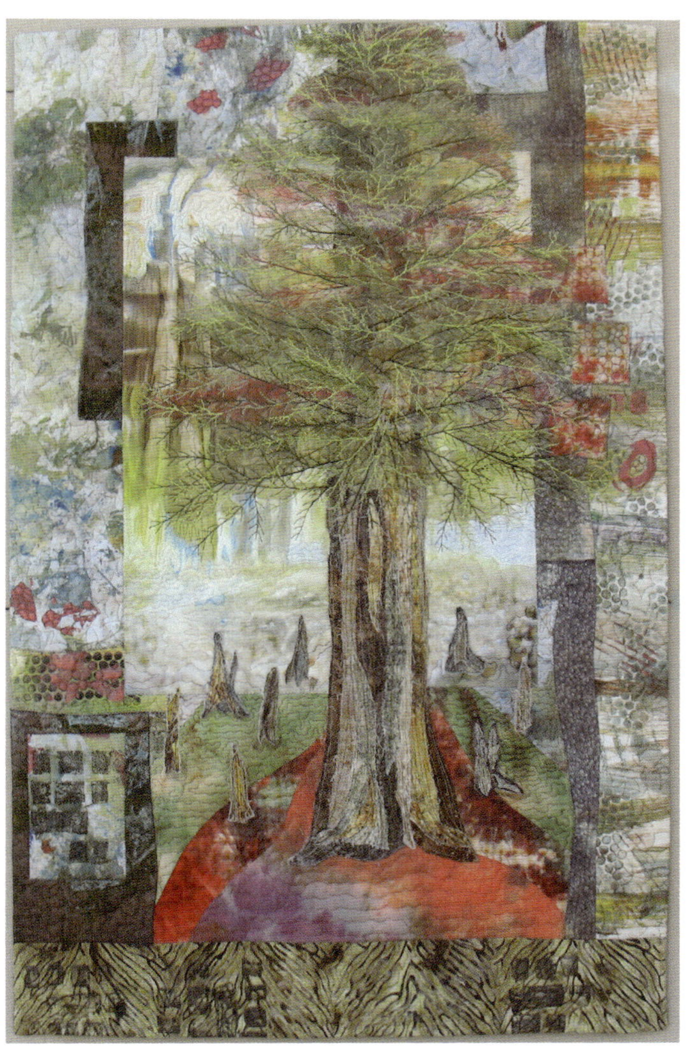

Judy Momenzadeh
Baton Rouge, LA, USA

Sentinel
22.5" x 34.25"

I am inspired by the trees around me, particularly the stately cypress. They are a very long lived tree and seemingly indestructible, always on guard in the natural world. They seem to me to be an allegorical symbol of God's angels, always on guard as well.

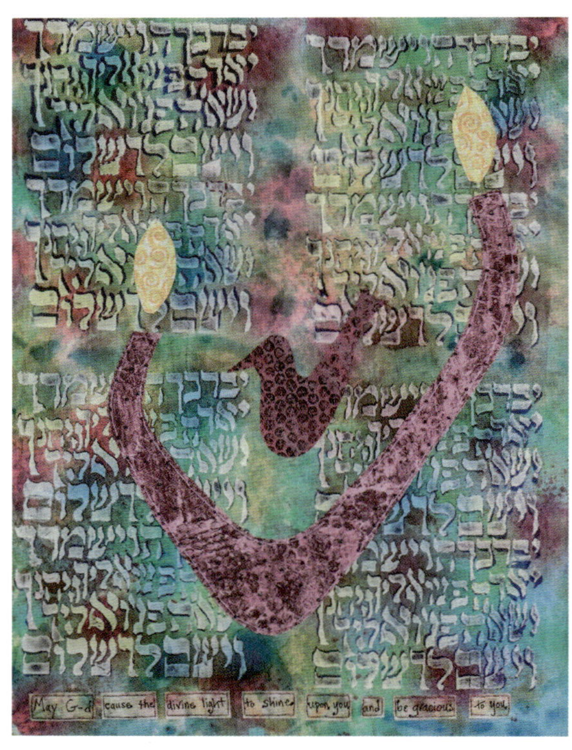

Susan L Robbins
Silver Spring, MD, USA

Shabbat Blessings
20" x 24"

Every Friday night for Shabbat, my mother would recite her blessings over the candles and put her hand on top of my head which is to make me feel special and loved. I didn't understand what these blessings meant since I am Deaf and I missed out the importance of the words. I was more fascinated watching the flickering flames. I am now using Judaic themes in my art work to enchance my learning within myself and signing the blessings which gives me the impact to understand them more. I try to instill myself to say the blessing for Shabbat: "May G-d cause the divine light to shine upon you and be gracious to you."

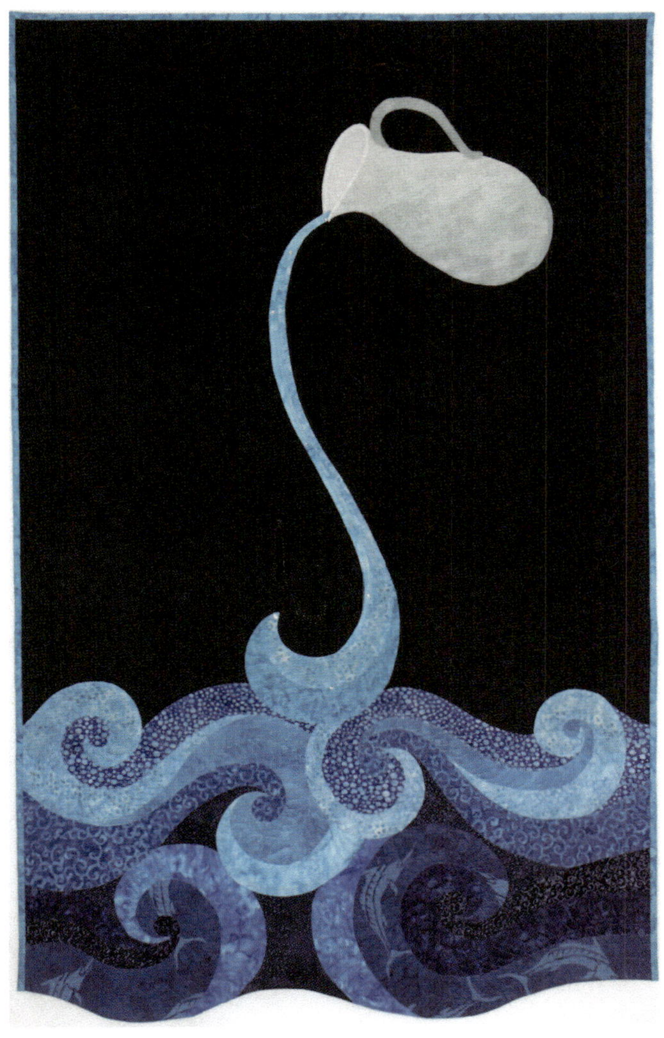

Amy K Johnson
Hurt, VA, USA

Poured Out 2
33.75" x 52"

Second in a series inspired by my church's logo, this quilt represents the feelings, good and bad, that I experienced during my husband's battle with cancer. Time and time again negative feelings threatened to choke my spirit, only to be conquered by a pouring out of love and grace that washed away the scary thoughts. At the same time, I was pouring myself out for my husband and children, one still an infant, and I was desperate to fill myself with the Living Water of God's love.

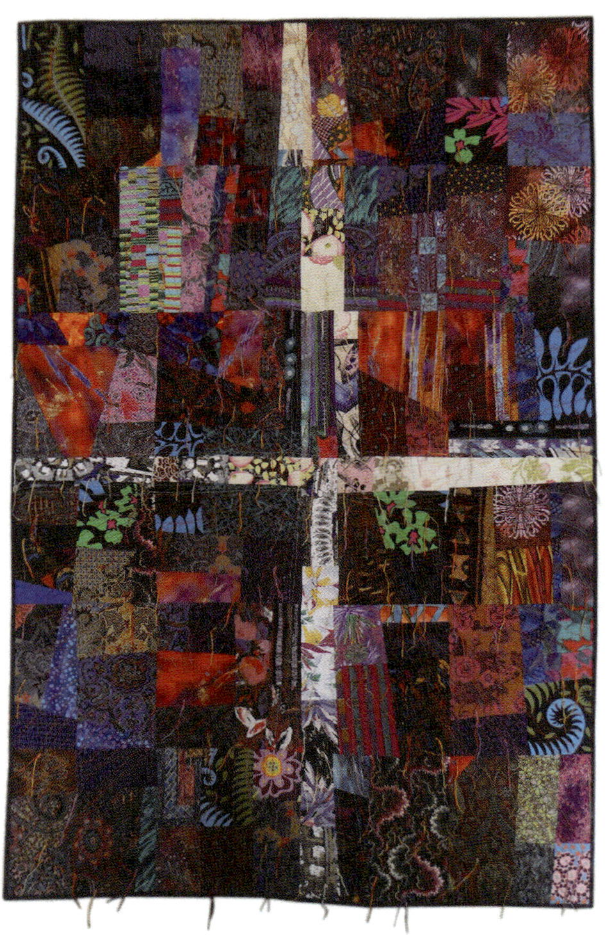

Diana F Sharkey-Leedy
Mount Kisco, NY, USA

Threads of Prayer

40" x 60"

The top was pieced two years ago. I began quilting in October 2012, titling it "Threads of Prayer." I was diagnosed with breast cancer November 2012. The quilting was completed in January 2013 just before my surgery.

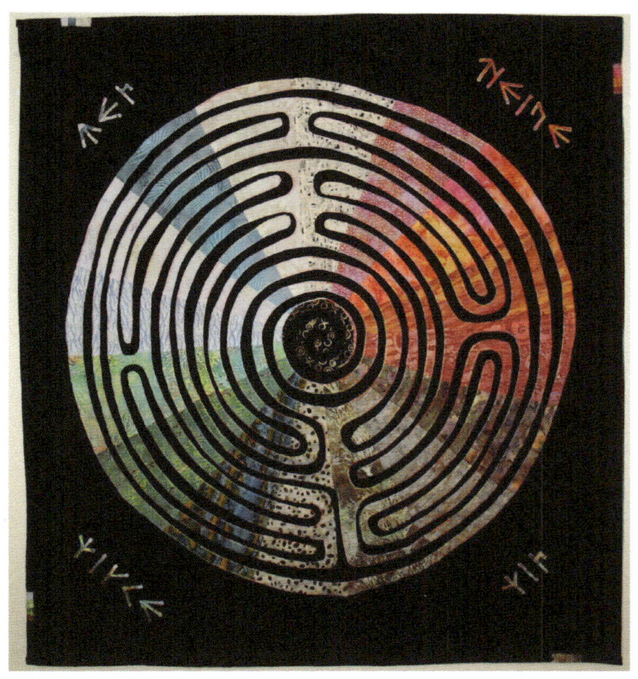

Debra Bentley
Xenia, OH, USA

Centering - Finding the Colors of My Soul
42.25" x 44.75"

This quilt was inspired by a walk in the outdoor, wildflower-planted labyrinth at the Marianist Environmental Education Center at Bergamo-Mt. St. John in Beavercreek, Ohio. As I walked through the labyrinth, shortly after my Mother's death, I experienced a sense of spiritual renewal and oneness with nature and my ancestors. Many religions use labyrinths and the classical elements as a basis for meditation and spiritual renewal. I chose to use the four classical elements of earth, air, fire and water to make the quadrants of the labyrinth and I labeled them with Old Irish Celtic Runes, for my Irish heritage.

AND I SHALL SEE THAT DAY
WHEN YOUR JUSTICE AND
POWER
WILL BREAK THE CHAINS
THAT BIND ME
AND MINE ENEMIES' LIES
STREWN
BROKEN AND EMPTY
YOUR MIGHTY HAND,
THAT AWFUL GRACE.
I WILL LIFT UP MY EYES
AT THE NAME
OF THE ONE WHO KNOWS ME
WELL.
(PSALM 63)

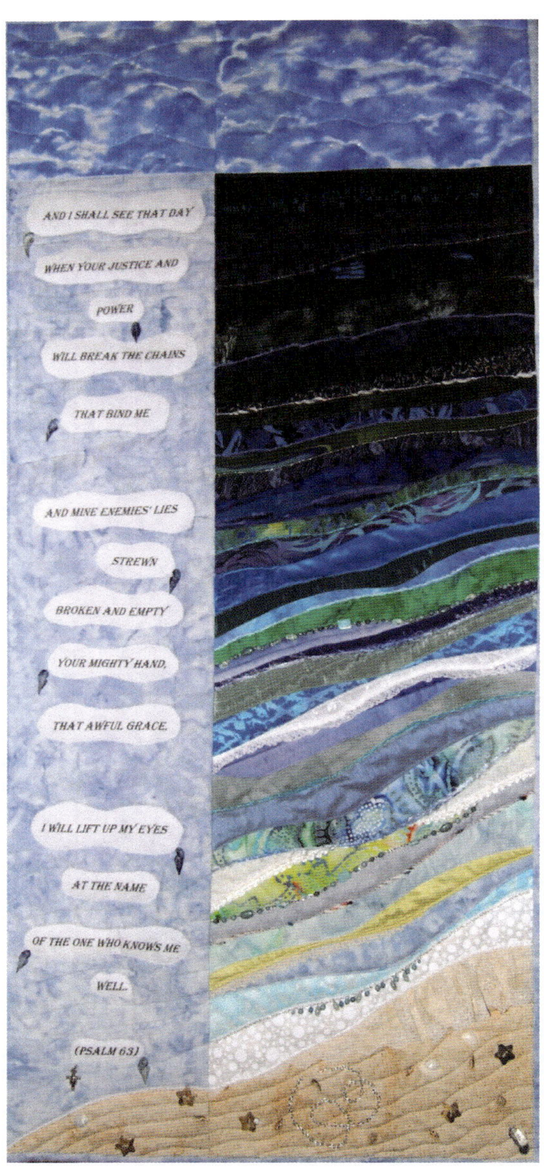

Nancy Firestone
Alexandria, VA, USA

Emergent Joy
23" x 50"

This quilt was inspired by the psalm I sing in my choir. The message of Psalm 63 and my faith helped me through a very difficult time of betrayal. I felt submerged in pain and sorrow but through God, family and friends I was able to break the chains and emerge into the light of hope, love and joy.

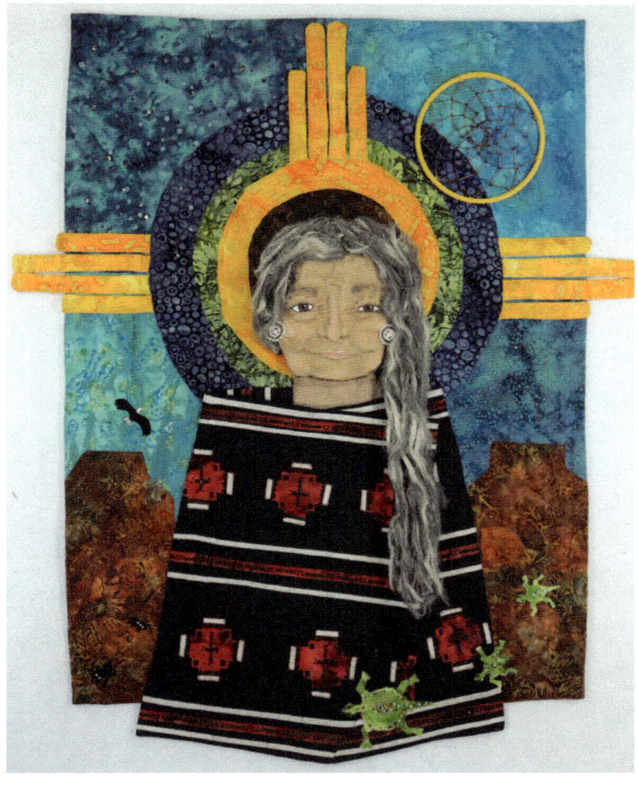

Nora Bebee
Rio Rancho, NM, USA

The Legend Keeper
34" x 40"

New Mexico is a magical land of history, cultures, and legends. Living here has brought a new sense of understanding and a deeper meaning to my life.I wanted to create a quilt that would be visual and emotional.

The quilt is filled with numerous symbols: seasons, compass points, Native American legends, the Zia, etc. The Legend Keeper, like all Grandmothers, was created to be the guide between the past and present. Viewers will be able to interpret and enjoy this quilt on many levels.

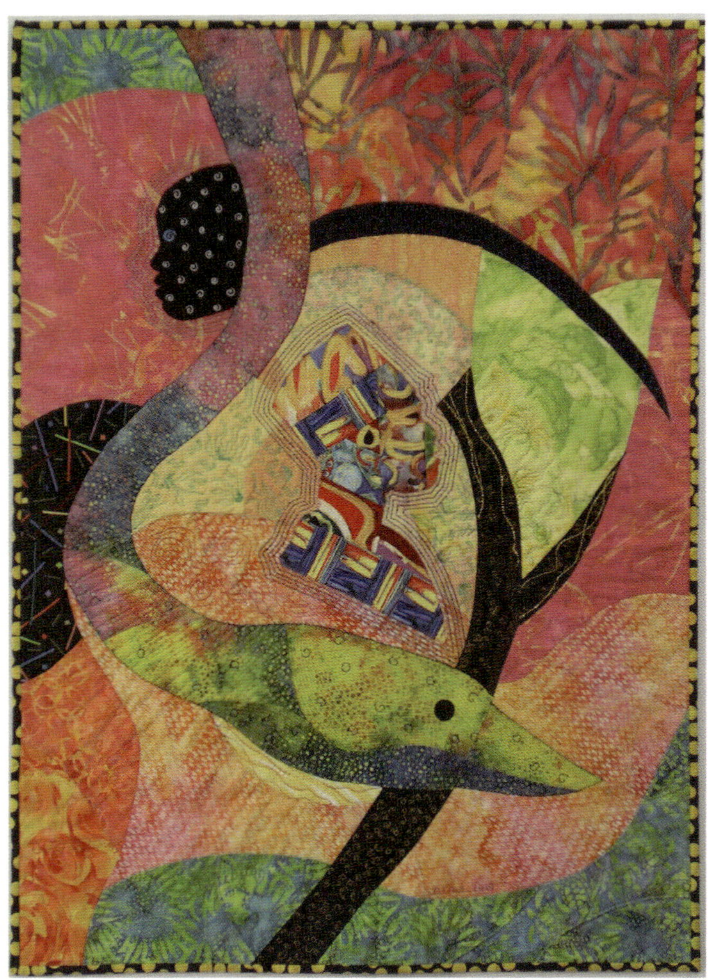

Lucinda Graber
Upland, CA, USA

What Snake?
28" x 38"

Tomorrow is my birthday! I will be 70 years old. I have gone deep into my soul to contemplate not only the meaning of My life, but the meaning of All life. "What Snake?" represents our human origin in the Garden of Eden. Older and wiser, I truly comprehend and celebrate that WE ARE ALL ONE, living togeher and sharing this holy universe.

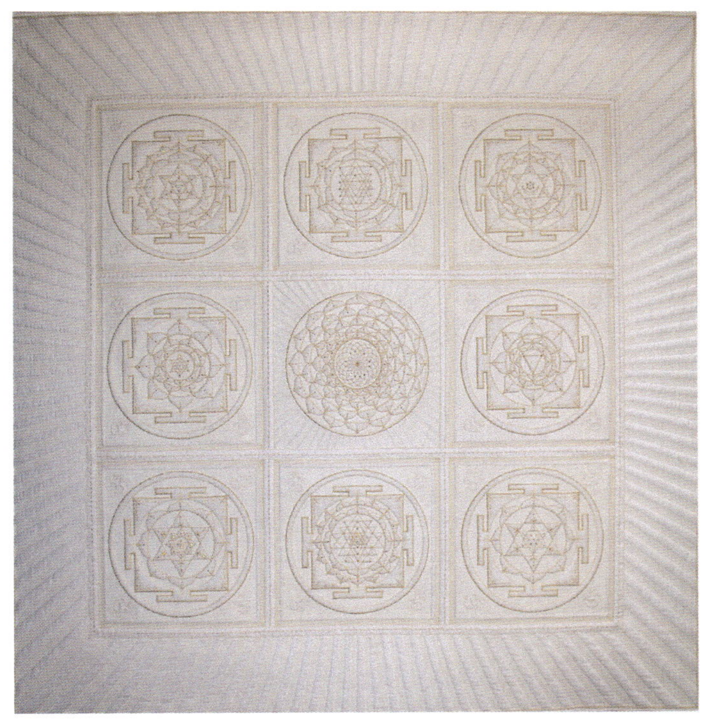

Pierra Vernex
Saint-Jérôme, QC, Canada

Simply Mandalas
90" x 90"

Simply Mandalas: a minimalist approach, dwelling zen spaces, and light and shadow contrasts rendering a chiseled marble effect from afar. Mandalas have always struck a familiar chord in me. Two things stand out in the journey of its making; how to attach an outer ray border to the 9 quilted/ assembled panels. Exploring other border designs to save myself the headache didn't work ; my mind kept sending me, loud and clear, the outer ray image, with mitered corners! I finally surrendered, trusted, listened, and the solution was there! The 7th chakra is often referred to as the 1000 petals crown (969 exactly). Imagine my surprise at counting afterward nearly 1000 individually decorative stitches! It felt like a wink from somewhere/somebody! Chuckling, I remember sending thanks back. Whenever my eyes rest on Simply Mandalas, serenity, peace and stillness fill me, and with a silent thanks, I smile.

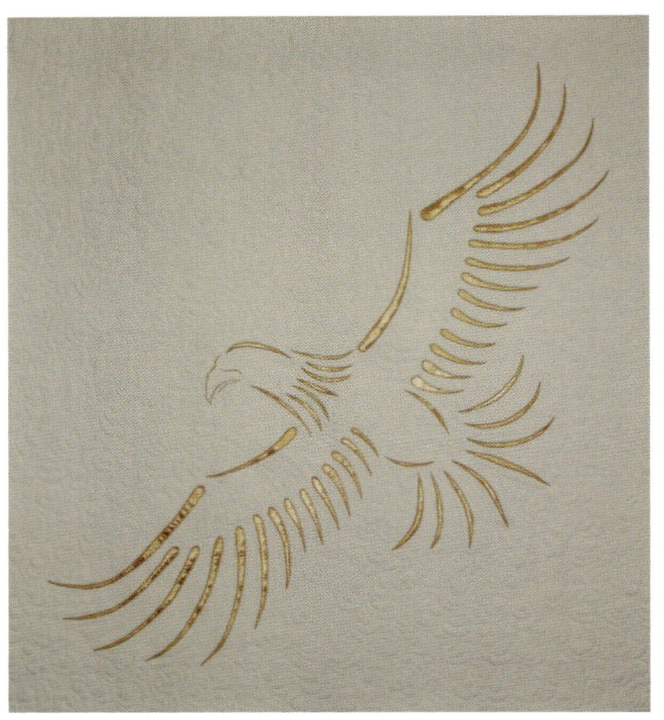

Susanne Meyer Fenelon Falls, Ontario, Canada
Soar on Wings Like Eagles 47" x 49.5"

This quilt is inspired by Isaiah 40:31. I have always been inspired by the majesty, strength and beauty of one of God's most magnificent creatures, the eagle. It is a great symbol of the freedom that God gives us to soar in our lives, if we accept the opportunities God presents to us.

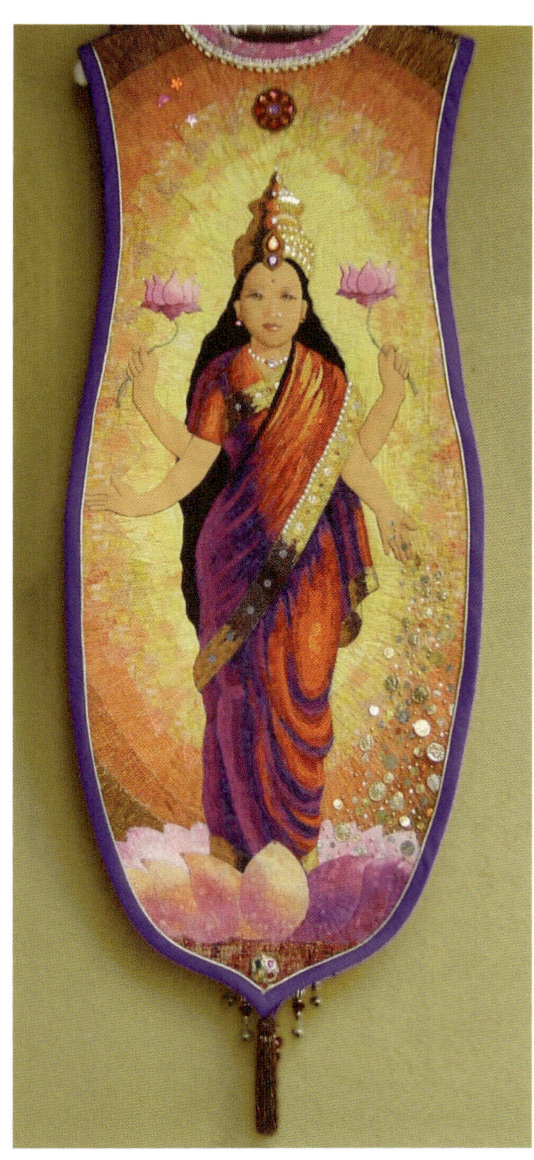

Meryl Ann Butler
Norfolk, VA, USA

Jewels of India: Goddess Lakshmi Tabard
16.5" x 46"

I consider the goddess Lakshmi (pronounced "Lock-shmee") to be one of the "jewels" of India. I created this tabard just before, during and after sharing my mother's sacred and amazing hospice journey. I find that focusing on the Divine Feminine in Her many forms always enhances my wellbeing. Lakshmi is the bestower of love, grace, light, beauty and abundance (both material and spiritual). Here, the color and value choices in both fabrics and threads create the illusion of three dimensions. I feel this contributes to making the essence of this goddess more palpable - to both creatrix and viewer!

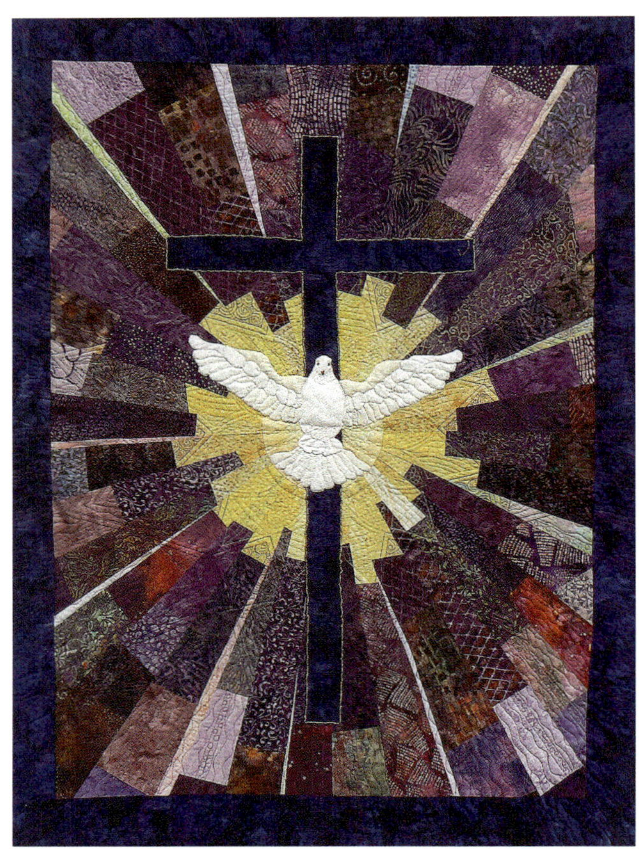

Jo Moury
Haymarket, VA, USA

Dove of Peace
34” x 44”

This is the first in a series of quilts depicting the birth, death and resurrection of Jesus Christ. Here, the Spirit of the Lord departs the cross as He makes the ultimate sacrifice for our sins. Radiating outward from the cross and dove is a quilted twelve pointed star representing the twelve apostles going forth to spread His word. Each of us is given gifts to share with others to the glory of God. Quilting is my gift and I love using this medium to both depict God's love for us and draw others to Him through my work.

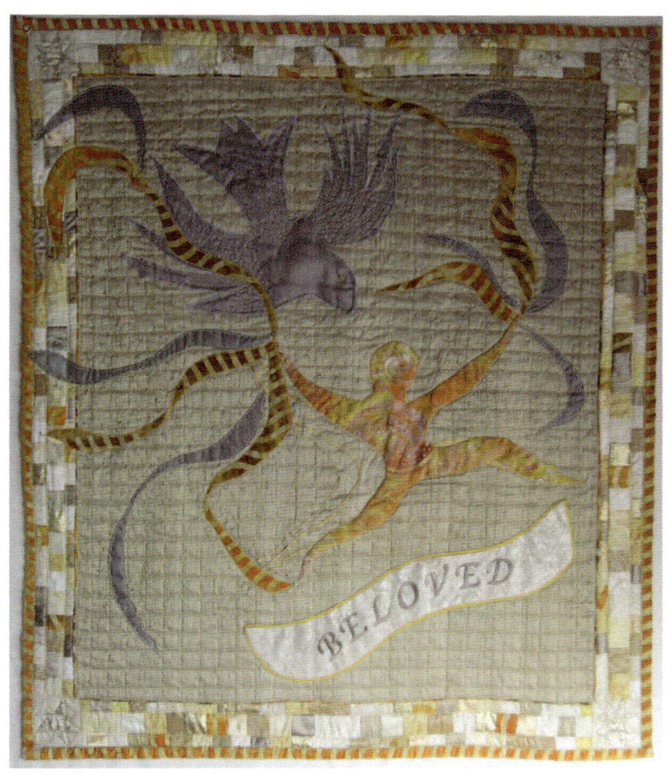

Marjorie Wilson Brooklin, ME, USA
Beloved 33.5" x 38"

Dance with abandon, leap for joy! "You are my beloved." Feel it, bask in it, let it fly! "You are my beloved." Know it, trust it, nurture it! "You are my beloved." Be astonished! These are the feelings I wanted to convey in this piece. Such a beautiful, healing , and joyful thing when we begin to know and love our true selves so that we may also know that divine spark which unites us all in love.

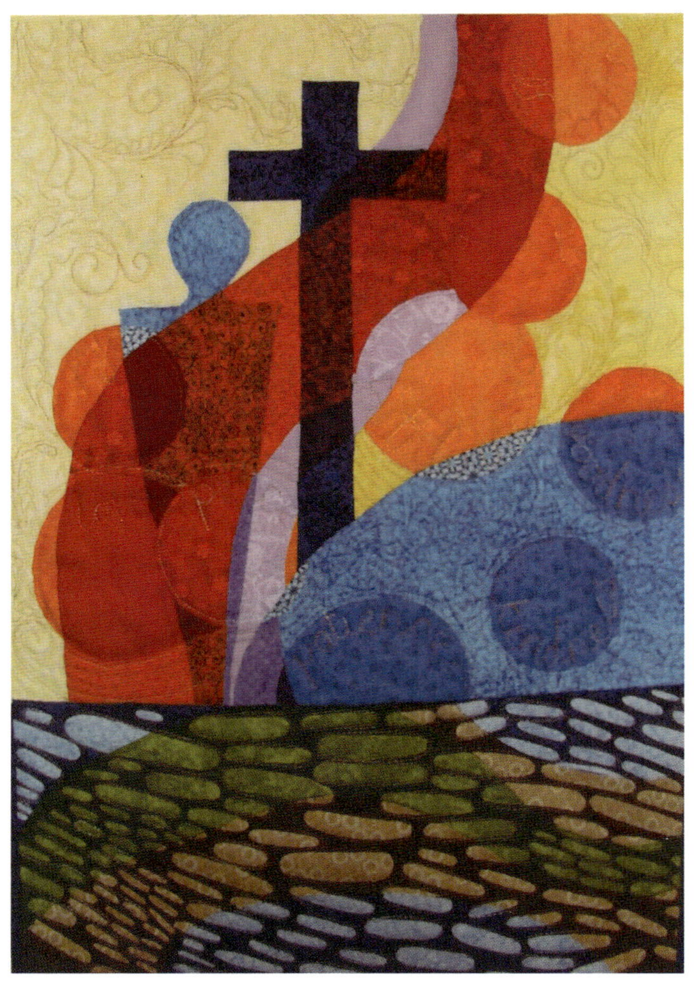

Susie Zolghadri
San Diego, CA, USA

His Guiding Spirit
21" x 30"

When my son Daniel was 15 years old he was confirmed and baptized. The passage from the Bible that he studied was Galations 5:22-23 (NIV). "But the fruit of the Spirit is love, joy, peace, patience, kindness, goodness, faithfulness, gentleness and self-control. Against such things there is no law." I was inspired to make an art quilt to celebrate Danny's confirmation. The bottom of the quilt represents our walk on earth. The main part of the quilt represents our walk of faith rising toward God, shadowed by the cross and guided by the fruits of the Spirit.

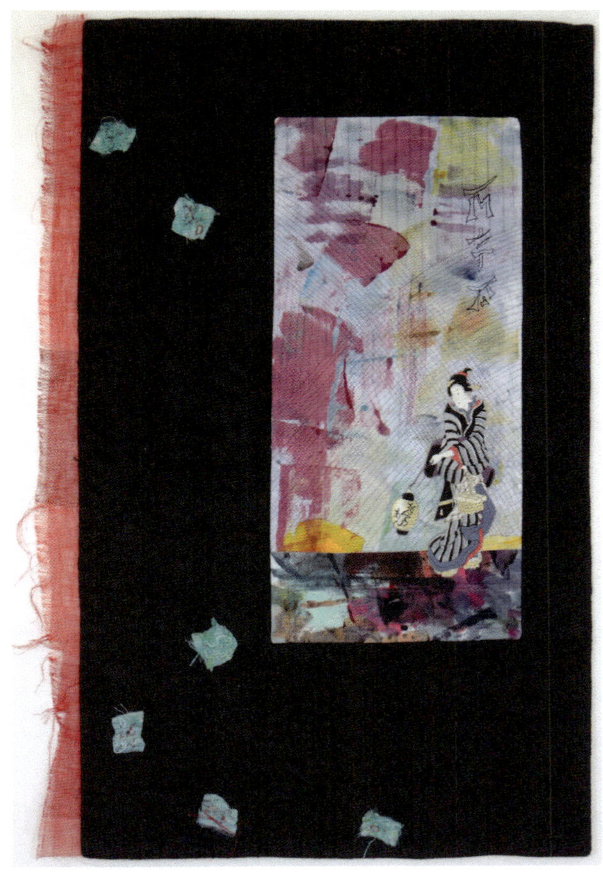

Meredith E Armstrong
Danville, PA, USA

The Seeker
21.5" x 32"

I often begin pieces with technical exploration. I wanted to combine a dying experiment with a new technique, trapunto. The woman with the lantern became the focus of my piece as soon as I saw her —she was looking for something, shining her lantern into dark water at dusk, seeing a glimmer of light below. The teal square of color became a reflection of her lantern, its glow like the soul's glow. I extended its shape and color over the dark field outside the central image, a whirling darkness from which we come and to which we return.

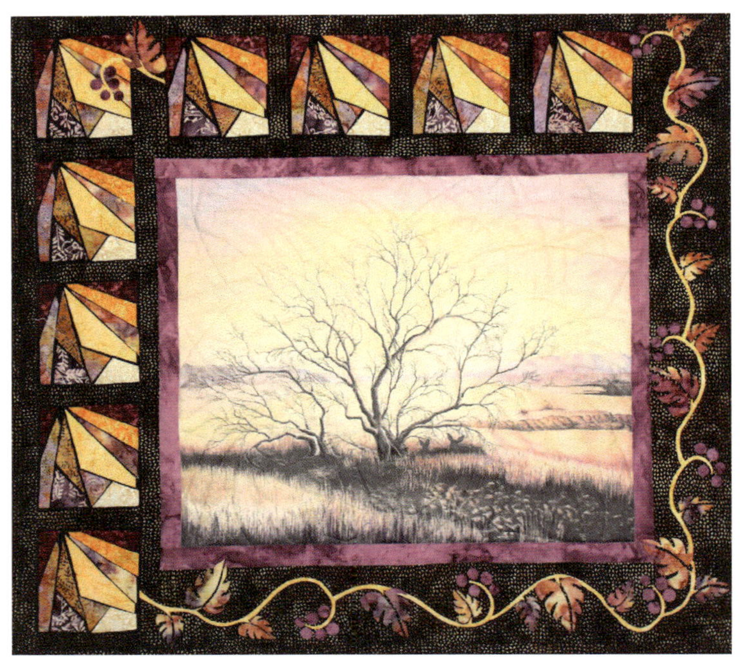

Gina M Gahagan Bozeman , MT, USA
Rest 35" x 31"

This quilt represents some of my recent reflections on life. We spend our days oganizing our lives and planning for the future. Even though we believe everything is "under control", events interfere with our plans. It is the sovereign Lord who is in control, and when things don't work out like we believe they should, He is still there for us when we seek Him. The quilt's border squares represent the order we want. The vines represent the constant presence of God, who is in control. The center represents the rest we should embrace no matter life's circumstances, knowing God is in control.

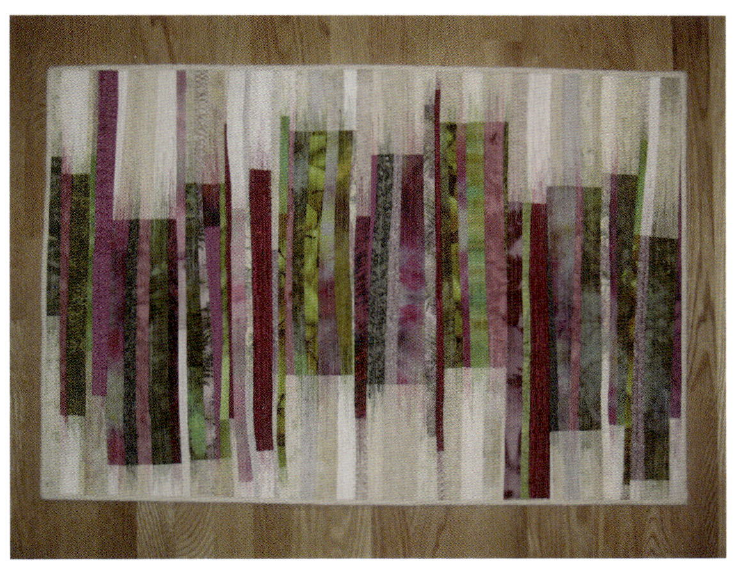

Christine L Thomas Madison, WI, USA
Side By Side 37.5" x 25"

Traditional liturgical colors morph, and life forms are glimpsed, expressing the nuanced spirituality and vitality of my church - a people stitched together as they work side-by-side rather than from positions of power. We honor the ancient Scriptural writings as solid building blocks for our lives (symbolized by blocks of strips), but recognize that each individual has unique insights into the Mystery we call God (expressed by strips that grow beyond those solid areas.) We're held in God's enlightening, transforming Spirit (shimmery creams.)
I offer this "heart work" in thanksgiving for the caring community of my newfound spiritual home.

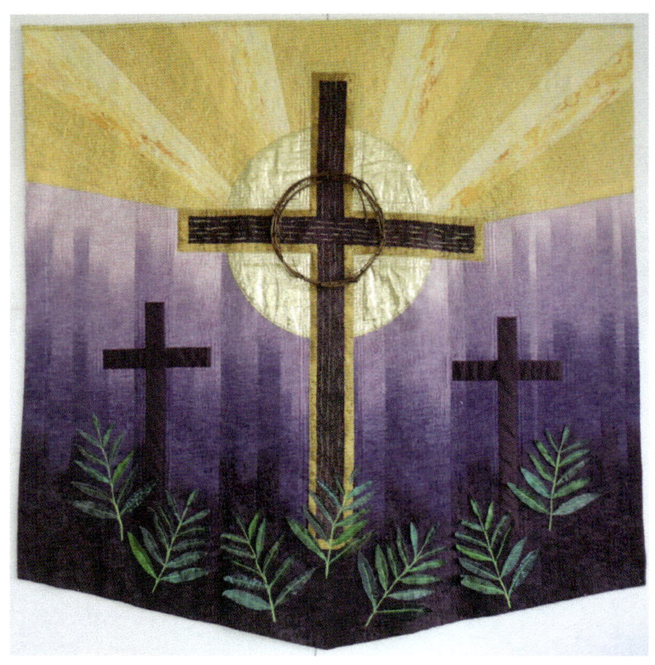

Nancy "Kay" Smith Belleview, FL, USA
The Journey Through Lent and Easter 55.5" x 54.5"

The Journey through Lent is a time of preparation for the celebration of Easter. This quilt has the following symbolism: "purple" is the royal color of kings and "palms" are traditionally waved to welcome the King. Jesus was crucified on the center "cross", the two thieves hung on the other crosses. The "crown of thorns" was placed on Jesus' head mocking him as a King. The "gold metallic circle" behind the cross and the "golden radiant sky" symbolize the resurrection of Jesus on Easter morning. Christians continue the Easter celebration by worshipping together every Sunday.

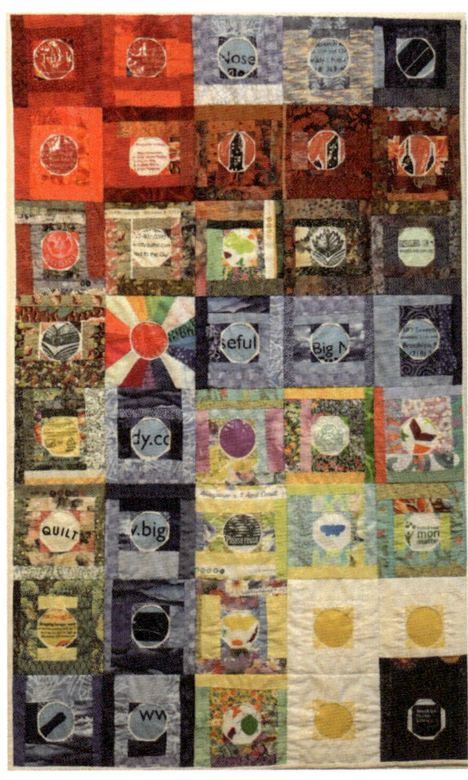

Valerie K Turer
Brooklyn, NY, USA

Green/Genesis: How Will It End?
27" x 43.5"

We tell stories about life on our planet, but the beginning and ending are unknown, and we understand only in part what is happening now.

This narrative reads lower right to upper left. - In the beginning, darkness covered the earth. "Let there be light!"The Lord God planted a garden in Eden. Rain fell forty days and nights. Rainbow sign: "Won't be water, but fire next time."

In the post flood world we see creation being destroyed. Pollution and extreme weather bring suffering to humankind. As the planet grows warmer will the "fire" bring about another flood, as the polar icecaps melt?

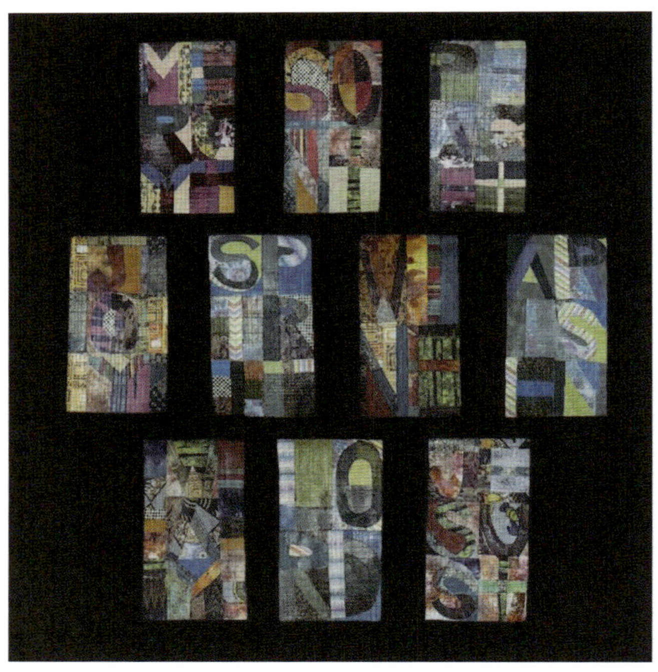

Susan B Callahan Silver Spring, MD, USA
Words of Inspiration 72" x 72"

This is a collection of 12 (out of a total of 20) quilted panels that hang in Good Shepherd Episcopal Church in Silver Spring, MD. They were inspired from an interactive sermon in June of 2011. All panels hang in especially designed niches in the Sanctuary.

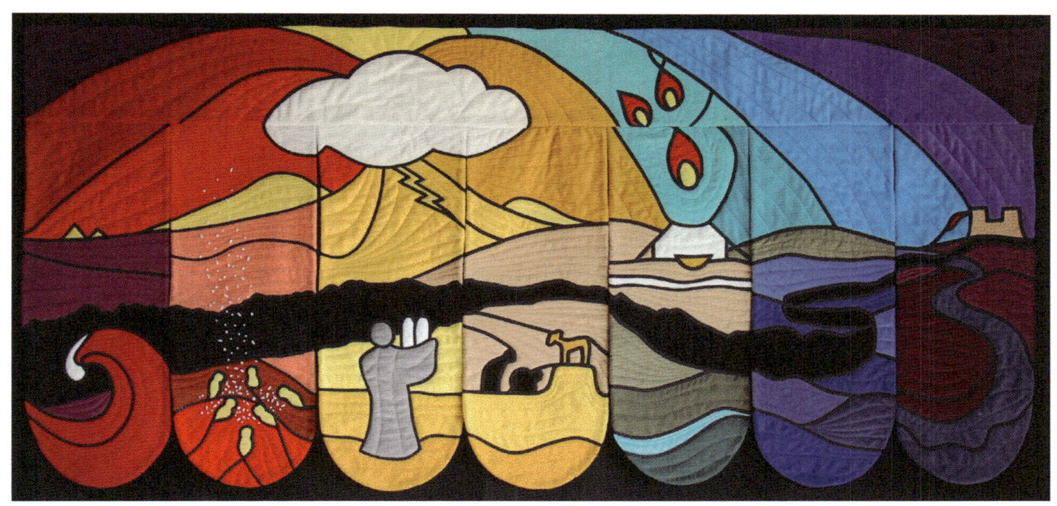

M C Bunte West Lafayette, IN, USA
Exodus 62" x 28"

The story of the Hebrew flight from Egypt to the Promised Land is a saga rich with examples of the human condition. It is symbolic of life's many highs and lows, inspirations, and lessons to be learned. In this work I selected seven important events from the journey—parting of the Red Sea, provision of manna and quail, the Ten Commandments, the golden calf, the Tabernacle, wandering for forty years, and eventually reaching Jericho. The cloud and pillar of fire in the sky evidence God's presence with them. I see this piece as a reminder of God's guidance and protection throughout life.

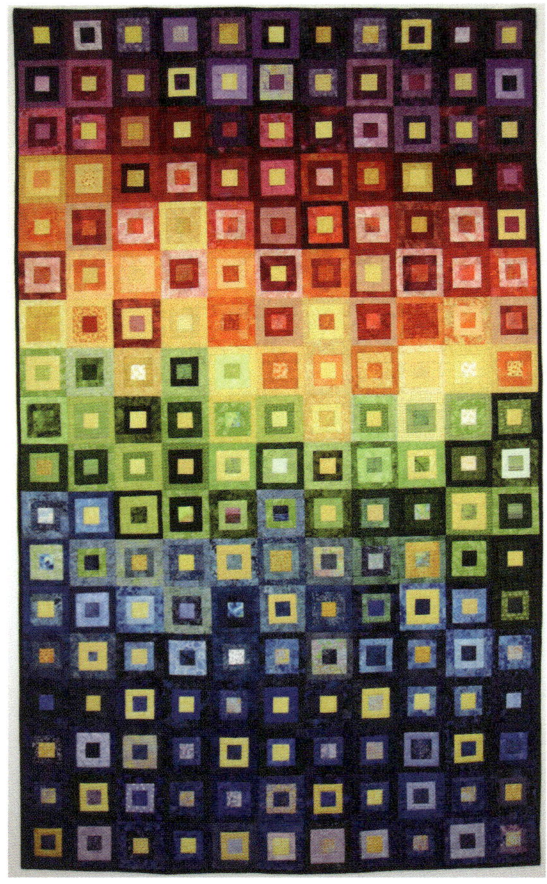

Kathryn Becker
Ashby, MA, USA

Grace in Full Color
47" x 77"

"We are each gifted in a unique and important way. It is our privilege and our adventure to discover our own special light." - Mary Dunbar

I've always been fascinated by light. Its energy at once warms, heals, surrounds and embraces us. It is a symbol for the all-encompassing energy that flows throughout the universe, connecting us with one another. When I imagined this quilt, I thought of how that light shines through us all, representing the unique talents and gifts that we bring to the world. I saw it shining brightly through windows of multicolored fabric.
Longarm quilted by Maureen Blanchard.

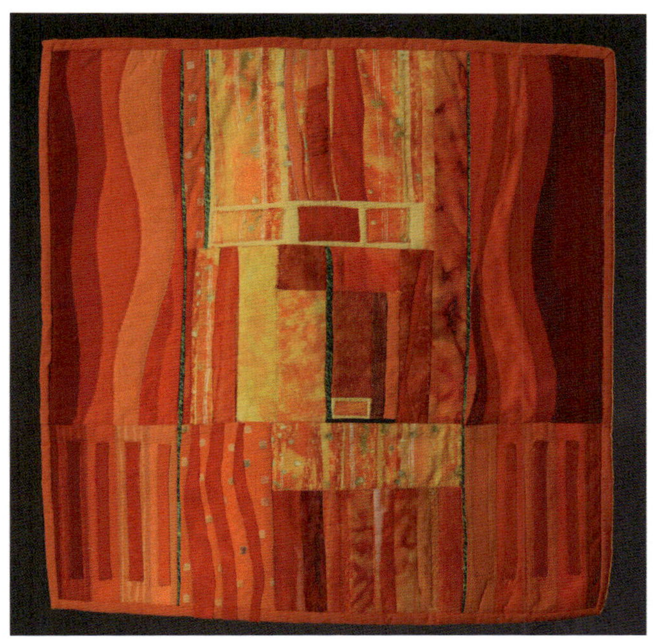

Linda H Hall Gahanna, OH, USA
Tending the Fire 24" x 24"

A growing relationship with God helps me confront the firestorms of life. We face many challenges throughout our lives. Our trust in God falters. Wants and wishes collide within the reality of our dilemma. Our reactions vary like degrees of heat. We might smolder, simmer or relate to the raging fire that destroys. When we are filled with the spirit of Christ, we physically and emotionally welcome God's power. The Holy Spirit is with us. My heartache will ease. I am once again trusting God to guide my journey.

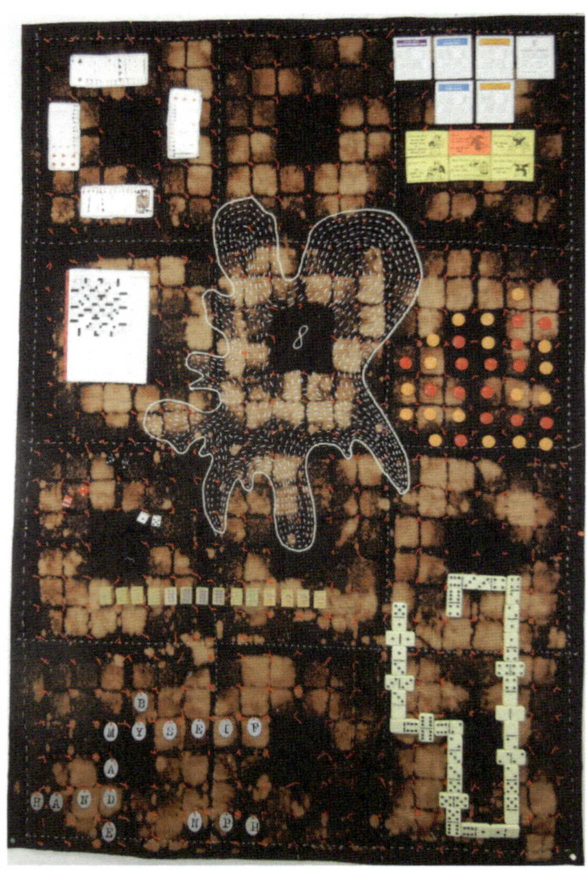

Nancy P Hicks
East Rochester, NY, USA

Is Life a Game or is there Something Else?
40 ” x 60”

In our fast paced, technology-driven world many people seem to feel technology is life. In actuality the world within each of us offers everything and more than they find superficially. Peace, guidance, joy, love and acceptance are available to each of us.

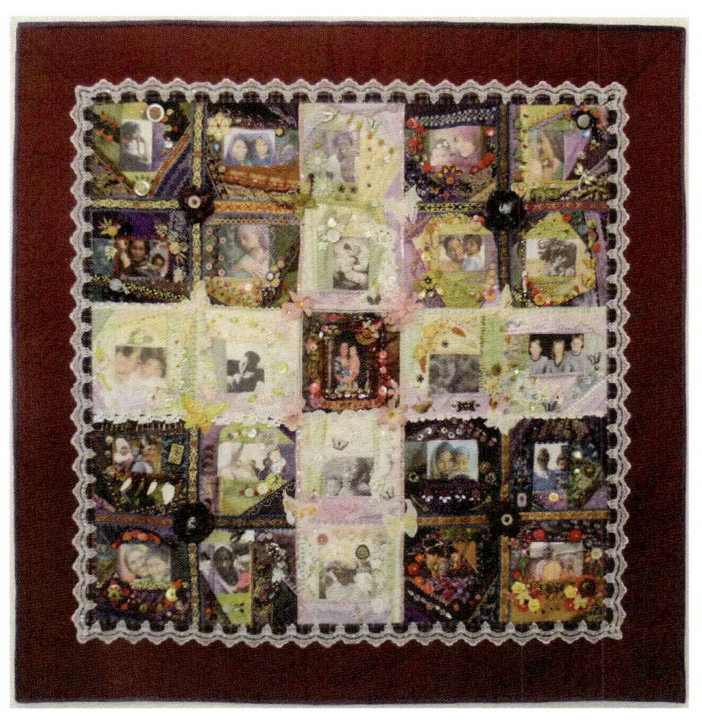

Debra L Spincic Montgomery, TX, USA
Mother and Child: My Mother, My Hope 57" x 57"

One evening while studying photographs of mothers I had an "Aha" moment! Each mother with their child was reminiscent of iconic Marian artwork. I designed this crazy quilt using many fabrics, stitches and embellishments to glorify these mothers in Her Image. While stitching, I felt a kinship with the mothers; sharing their immediate joys and understanding their future sorrows. Each mother became the Virgin Mother; a mother filled with love and sorrow for her child.

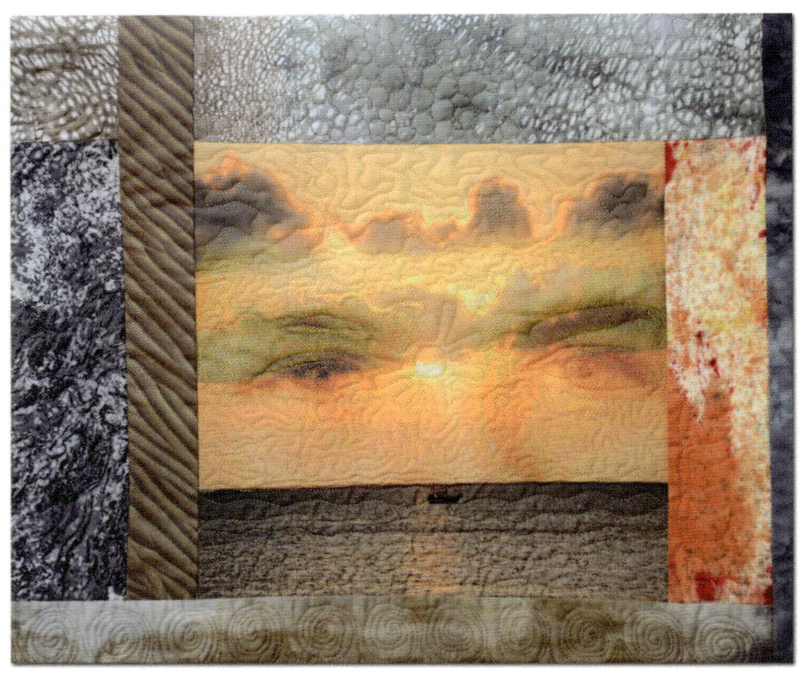

Bonnie D Askowitz Miami, FL, USA
Lookin' Down on Creation 20.75" x 17.25"

"Lookin' Down on Creation" is about women as Creator. Women.create from birthing to the creation of full lives for our families. We also create through the making and recording of history through visual art, music, and storytelling. My idea of the Spirit is feminine, like a mother. She is "Lookin' Down." What does she see? Does she see love? I think so. Does she see hate? I am afraid so. Does she see waste and greed? Oh, yes. But still she sees optimism and she sees hope.

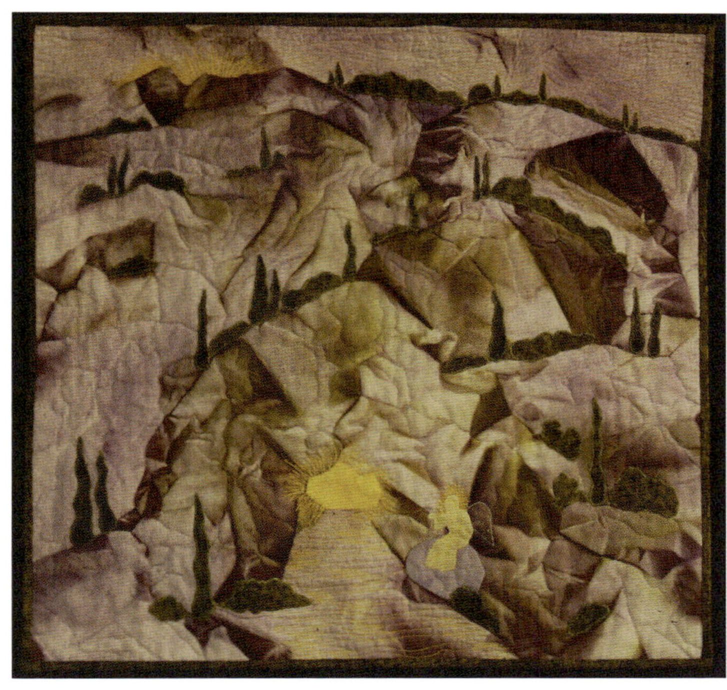

M C Bunte
West Lafayette, IN, USA

On the Third Day
21" x 20"

Often my artistic ideas are inspired by experiences and events of those around me, but this work came about in a different way. One day I was looking through a stash of fabrics that I had air-brushed and was struck by how one piece resembled rocky hills. As I rotated the cloth a cave seemed to emerge, reminding me of the terrain surrounding Jerusalem. Instantly I thought of Christ's tomb and the miracle of His resurrection! What would the first visitors have seen when they arrived there in the early morning? It was a reminder of the hope for eternal life/perpetuity found in most religions. The resulting scene also reminds me of late-medieval paintings that used stylized landscape forms and symbolic nimbuses.

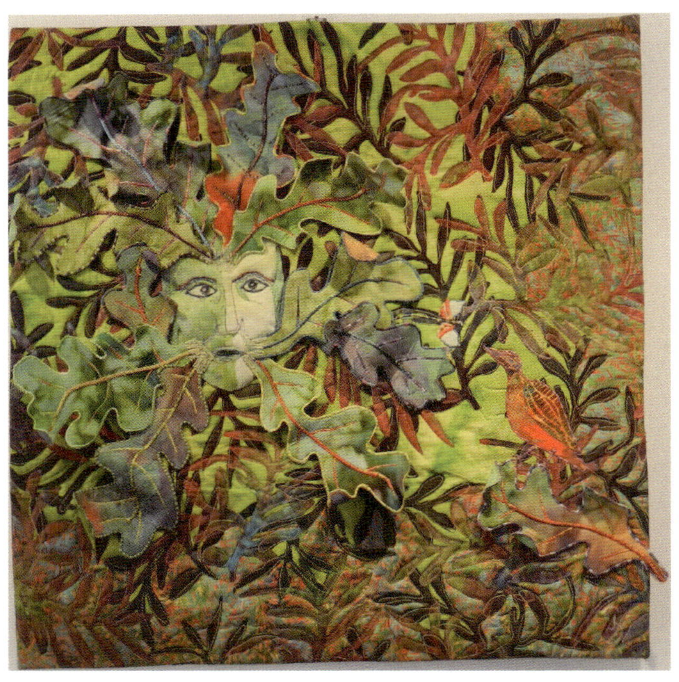

Joan Stogis Silver Spring, MD, USA
Green Man 24" x 24"

The Green Man represents to me the irrepressible vitality of life, and our oneness with the earth. I am drawn to his image again and again. A pre-Christian figure, he is frequently found in medieval cathedrals, whence I have derived my inspiration.

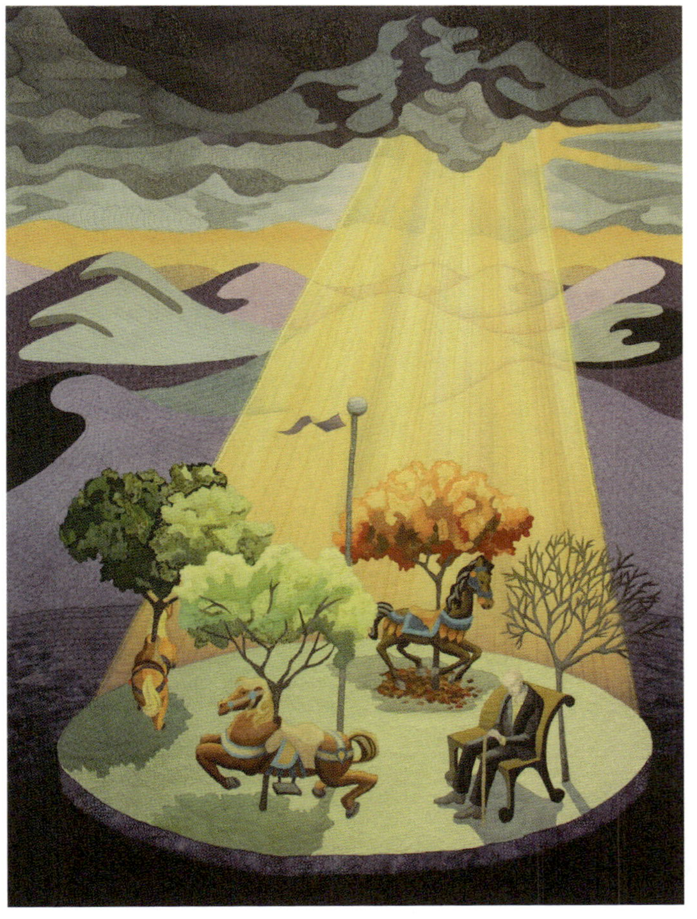

Linda Anderson
La Mesa, CA, USA

Carousel of Time
46" x 58"

"And the seasons, they go 'round and 'round, and the painted ponies go up and down. We're captive on a carousel of time..."--Joni Mitchell.

I have been inspired by these words for decades. They so beautifully and hauntingly express this journey called Life we all ride. Some of us leave early, others ride until we can no longer climb upon the horse. But we all return to the shining light behind the roiling clouds.

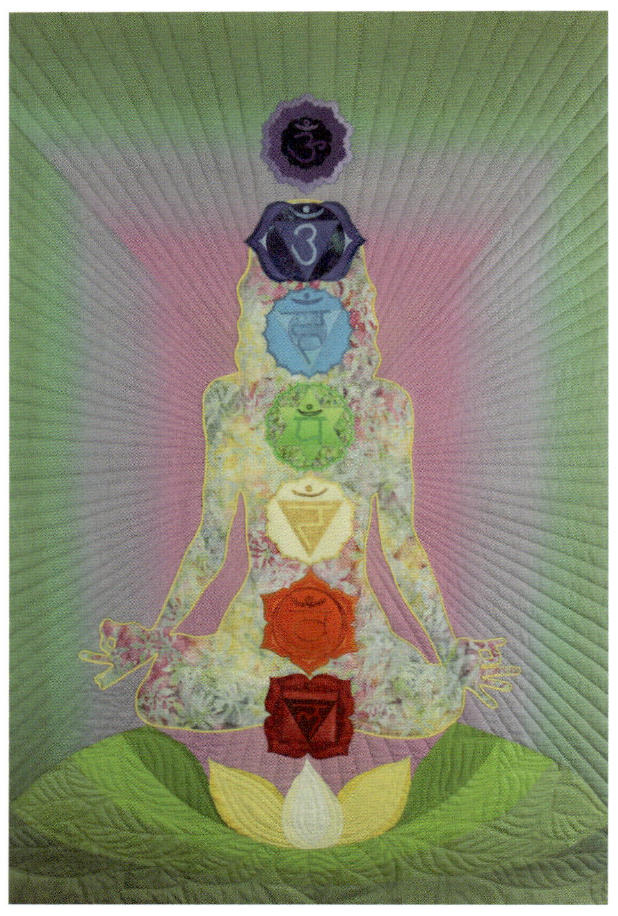

Doris A Lovadina-Lee
Toronto, Ontario, Canada

Radiant Light
54.5" x 68.5"

This quilt embodies the divine life force in women. Chakra centers correspond to seven centers of energy in the human body. These spiraling wheels of vibrational energy channel power into and out of the body. When this vital energy flows easily we remain in physical, spiritual and emotional alignment. The portrayal of the chakras superimposed on a female figure honours this divine/vital/transformative power. This quilt is a reminder to us all to be nurturing of ourselves, to be present in the moment, and to be in tune with the creative life force within us.
Longarm quilted by Sandy Lindal.

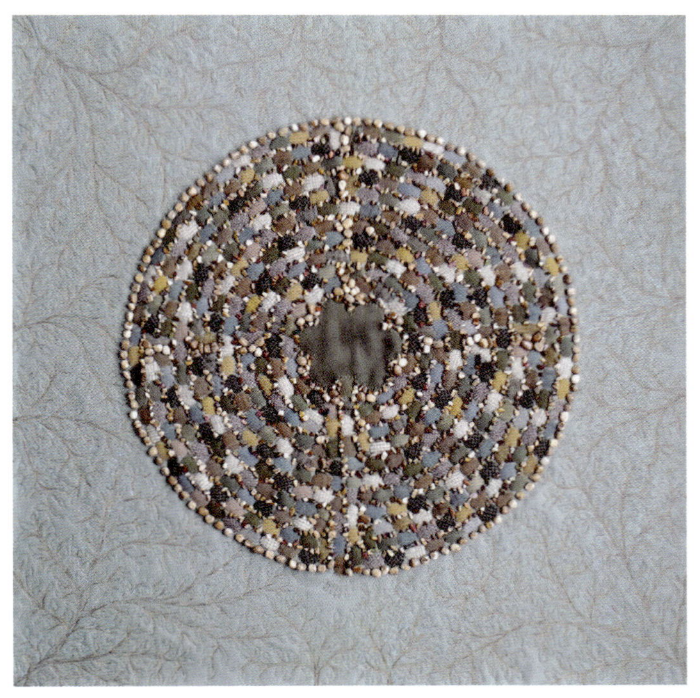

Sarah Entsminger
Ashburn, VA, USA

Lord, Hear My Prayer 34” x 34”

Walking a labyrinth is an incredibly spiritual journey for me, a place where I can feel the Lord's presence as he walks with me. I will often focus my thoughts with a Taize chant. This quilt was created to be experienced in spiritual meditation by those unable to walk a labyrinth. Your finger follows the wool pavers kept gently on the path by the pebbles to the center to linger for prayer and contemplation before following the path back to the entrance. My favorite labyrinth is located in the woods beneath towering trees at Shrinemont in Orkney Springs, Virginia.

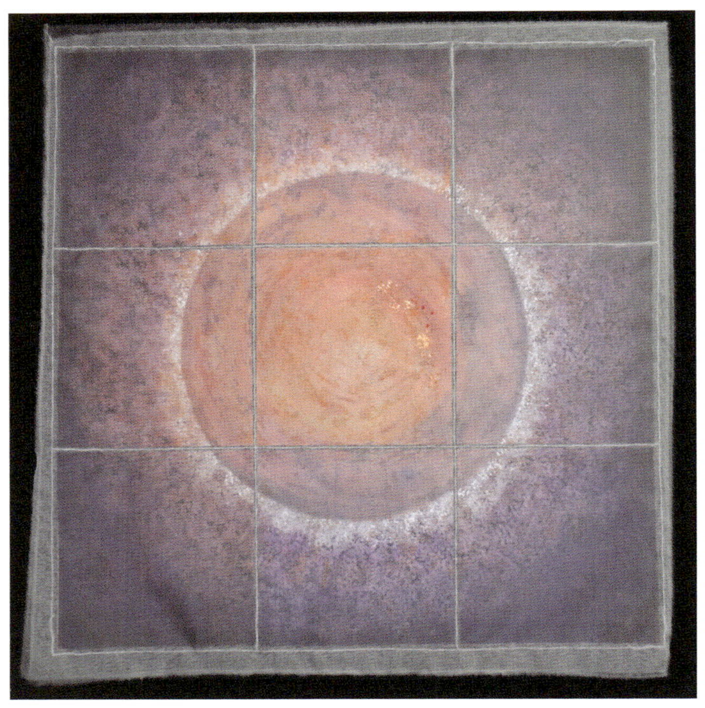

Lisa Kerpoe San Antonio, TX, USA
Origins 24" x 24"

My recent work is focused on creating a sense of luminosity. I am fascinated by the use of color, value and contrast to make a piece glow and come to life. My goal with Origins is to represent the light of Spirit that lies within and is the source of all.

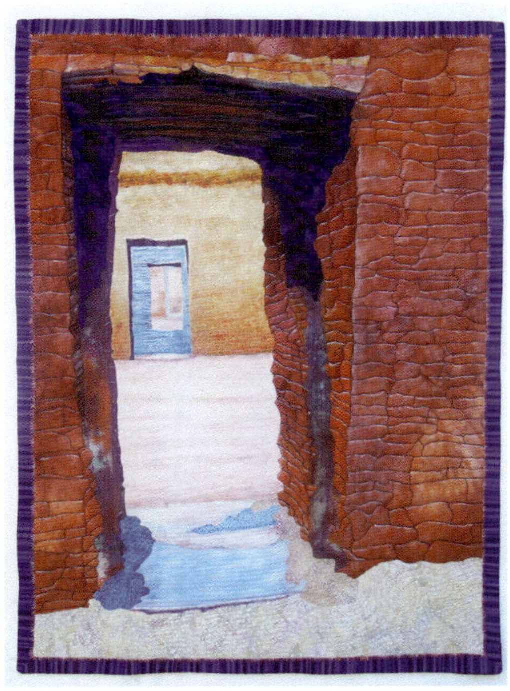

Sally G Wright Los Angeles, CA, USA
Chaco I 27" x 37"

This series of doors in the Pueblo Bonito at the ancient Anasazi native American site at Chaco Canyon in the Four Corners area of New Mexico fascinates the visitor and draws one deeper and deeper into another world of mysteries. The idea of discovery drew me in - wondering what revelation I might find as I entered one sacred space after another on my own spiritual journey.

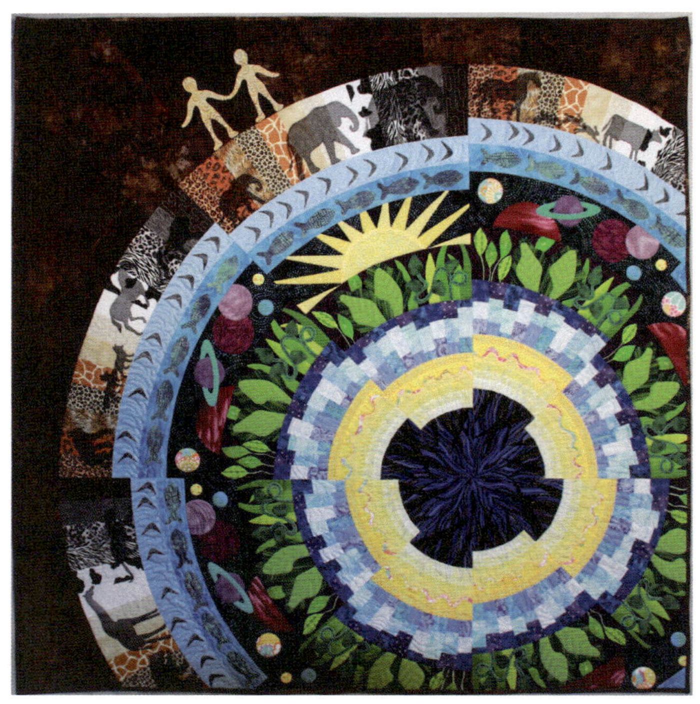

Linda Evans Murrieta, CA, USA
In the Beginning 56" x 56"

This piece is an homage to the greatest Artist who ever existed and His amazing creation. You can read all about it in the first chapter of the Bible.

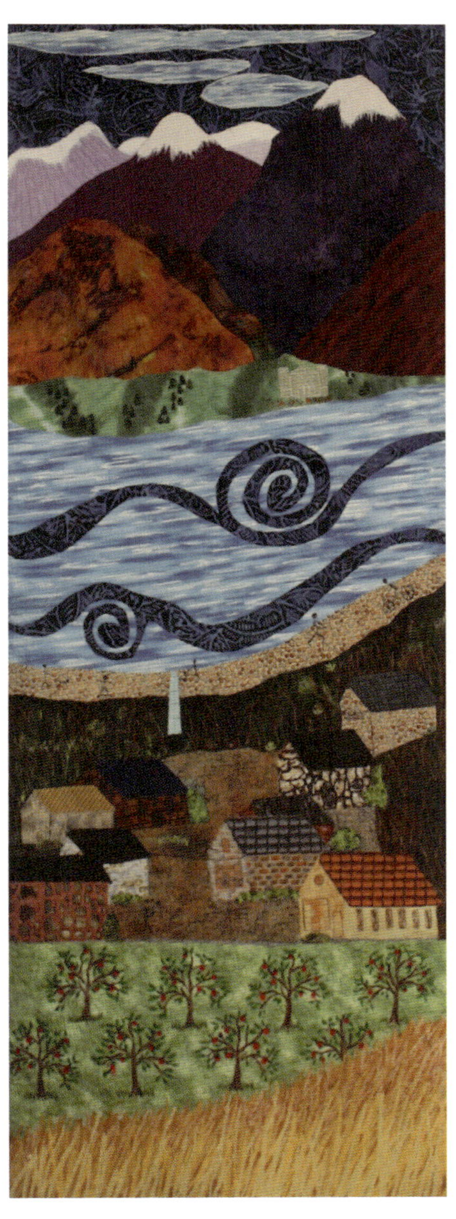

Denise (Denny) C Webster
Simpsonville, SC, USA

ArtQuiltRivers-Boulder
20” x 60”

The first time I saw the Boulder Valley I experienced Chief Niwot's curse - to be destined always to return to this beautiful place. Purple mountains, amber waves of grain, spacious skies filled my heart to bursting.

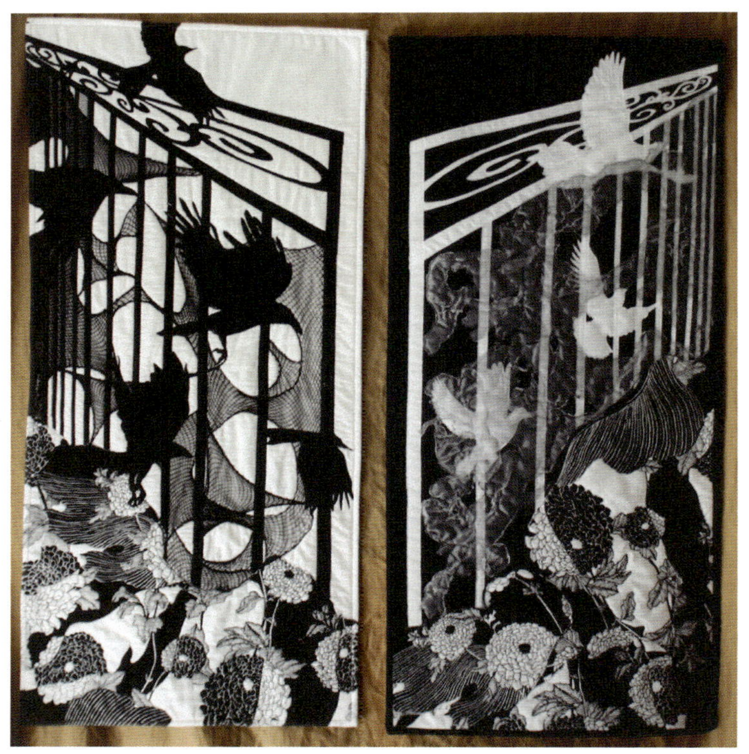

Stacy Hurt Orange, CA, USA
Gates of Heaven and Hell 42" x 42"

This piece explores the common perceptions of heaven and hell and has a discussion with the viewer of the paradox between the two by use of color, texture and placement.

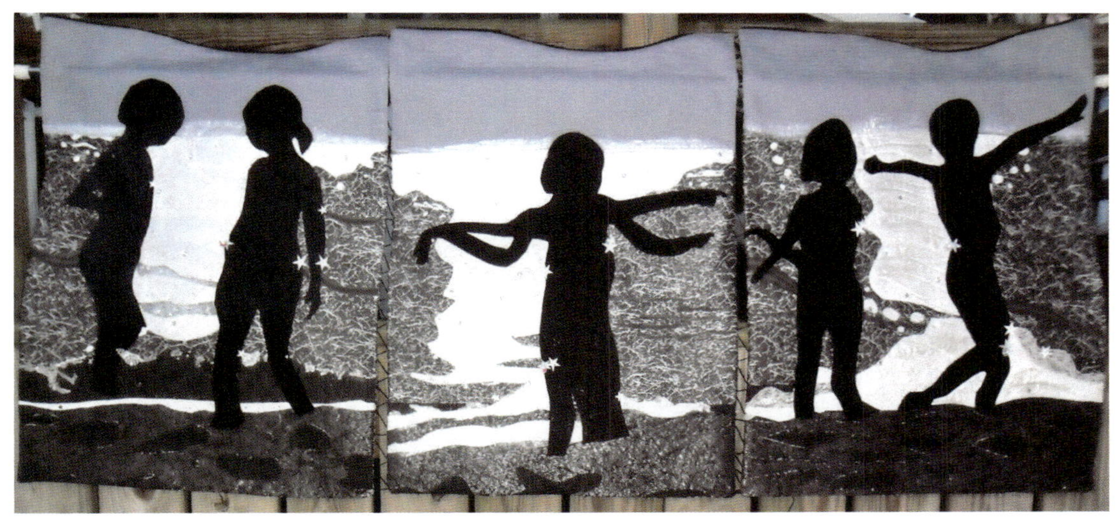

Dolores M Johnson Huntington, WV, USA
Holy Encounter 68" x 20"

"When you meet anyone, remember it is a holy encounter." This quotation from A Course in Miracles always reminds me that we are ONE in holy moments. In 2010 my friend Beth Darby, an amateur photographer, took pictures of her grandgirls on a moonlit beach. I could hardly wait, after she gave me permission, to make this quilted triptych, which so graphically illustrates ideas I deeply hold.

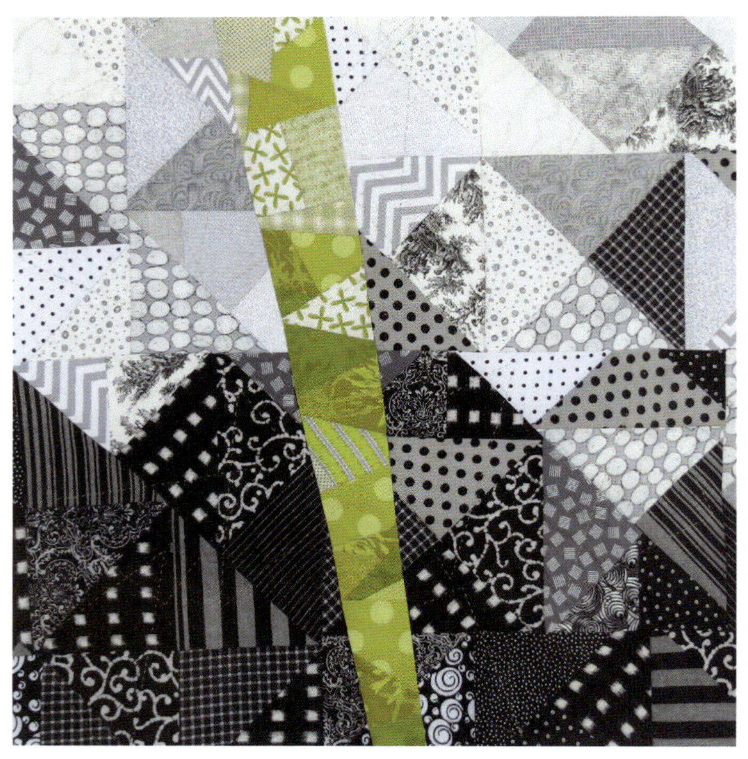

Joanell Connolly Huntington Beach, CA, USA
That's How the Light Gets In 43" x 43"

"That's how the light gets in" reflects an event that occurred while dealing with pain and feeling profoundly alone. What occurred brought peace and changed my life. The title is borrowed from Leonard Cohen's poem "Anthem." The chorus concludes with, "there is a crack in everything; that's how the light gets in."

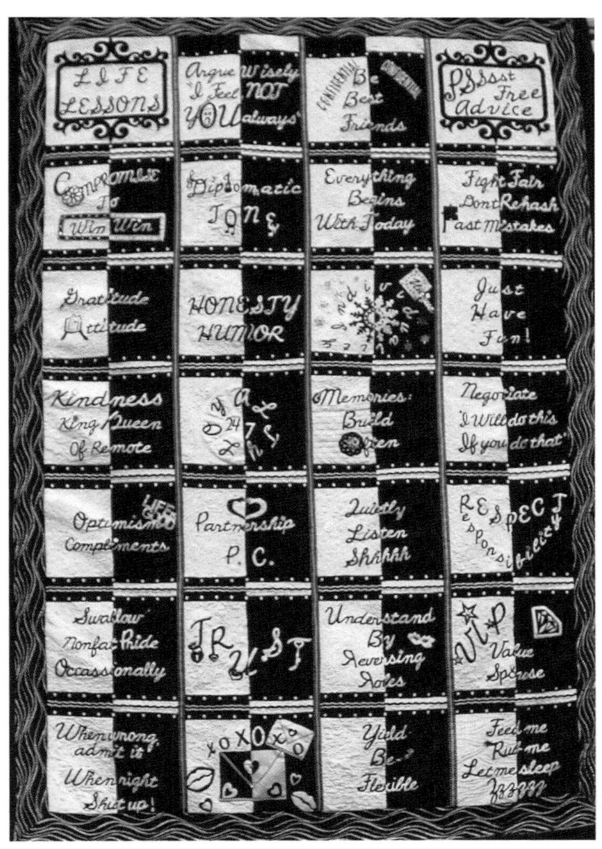

Meena Schaldenbrand
Plymouth, MI, USA

Marriage, Life Lessons & Free Advice For My Daughters!
51" x 69"

Argue Wisely... Say "I feel", not "You Always"... Be Best Friends... Compromise to Win/Win... Diplomatic Tone... Everything Begins with Today... Fight Fair... Don't Rehash Past Mistakes... Gratitude Attitude... Honesty... Humor... Individuality... Kindness... King/ Queen of Remote... Loyalty... Memories: Build Often... Negotiate: I will do this if you will do that... Optimism... Partnership.. P.C... Quietly Listen... Respect... Responsibility... Swallow Nonfat Pride Occasionally... Trust... Understand by Reversing Roles... VIP. Value Spouse... When wrong, admit it. When right, shut up!... X O ... Yield: Be Flexible..."Feed me, Rub me, Let me Sleep ZZZ"

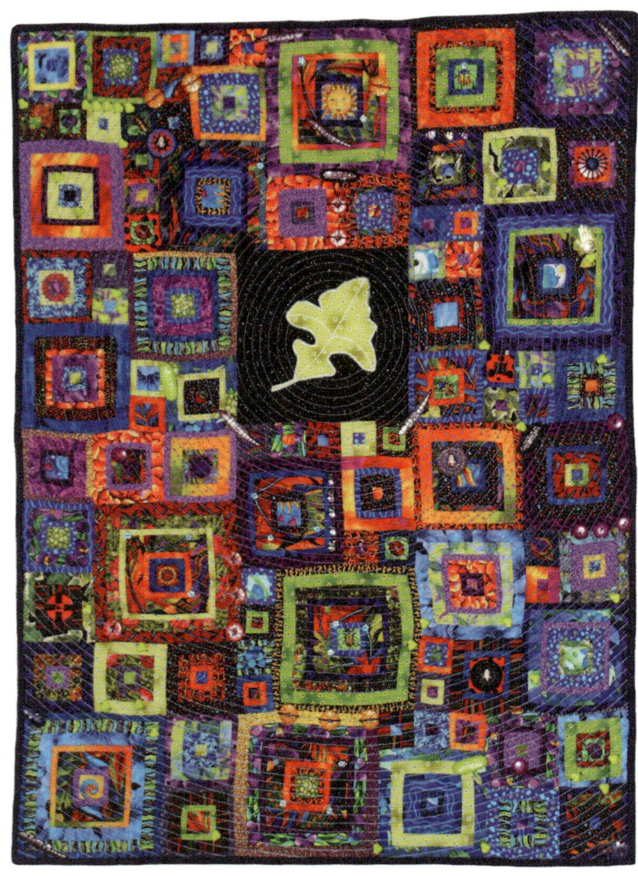

Lisa Binkley
Waunakee, WI, USA

The Quiet Place
26” x 36”

The world, with all of its beauty, can also feel loud and overwhelming. We all need a quiet place—ideally found within ourselves—in which to calm our minds and center ourselves, so that we can go back out into the world and peacefully go about our work and lives.

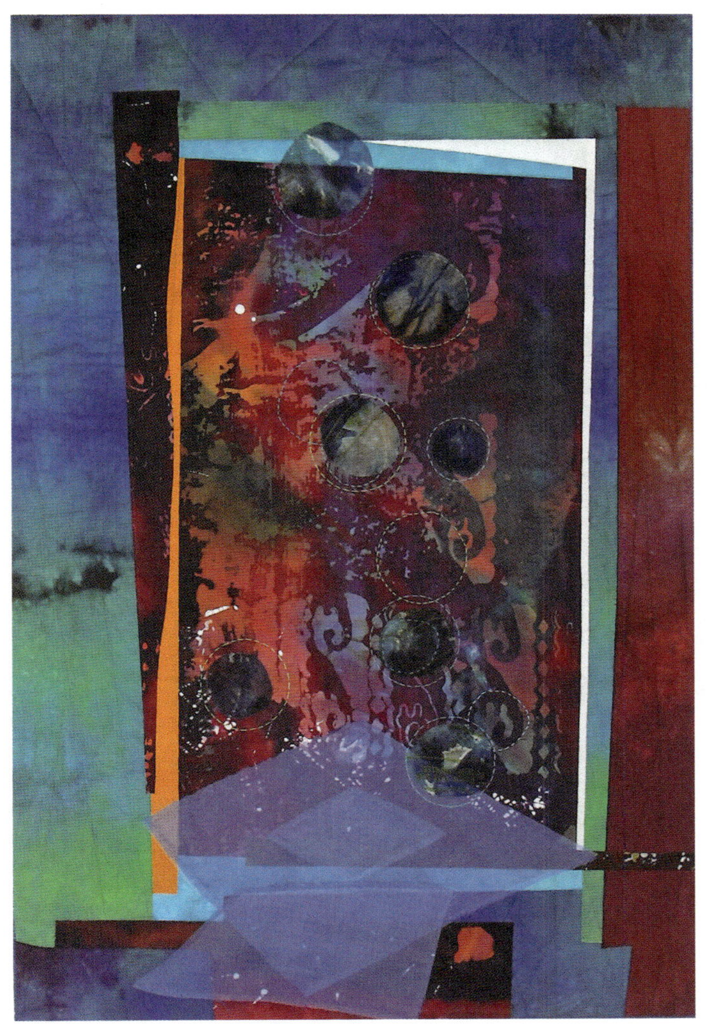

Dianne V Dockery
Kutztown, PA, USA

Prayer Closet III
25" x 36"

This piece depicts a deliberately allocated berth where prayers ascend and the voice of God vibrates deep into my spirit. My prayer closet is a sacred space for God's presence.

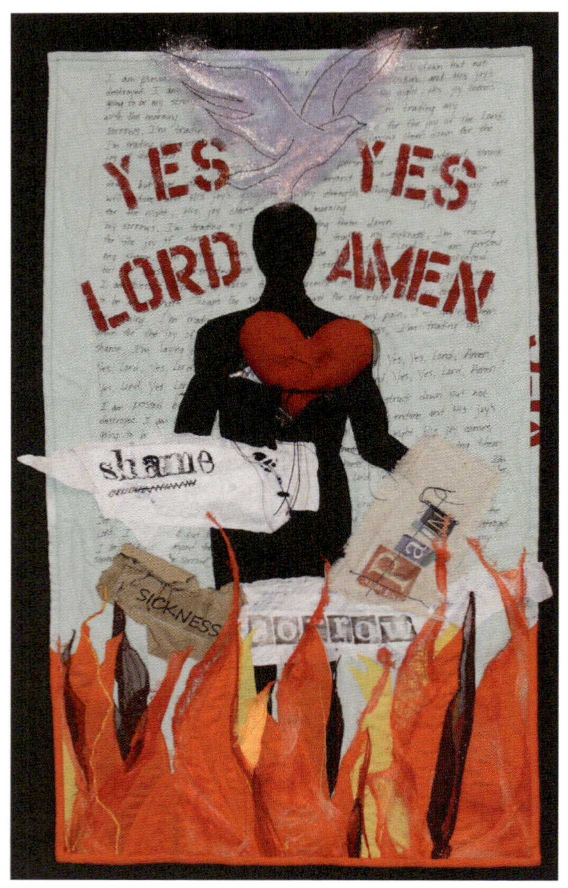

Lori East
Carthage, MO, USA

Trading My Sorrows
18” x 30”

The greatest joy in my life is my relationship with Jesus. That He could love me, in spite of me, just astounds me. The blessings He gives me, blessings I don't deserve, amaze me.

This quilt was inspired by my love for a song that explains that joy better than any words I have.

"I'm trading my sorrows, my pain, I'm laying them down for the joy of the Lord." The chorus, "Yes, Lord, Yes, Yes, Lord," translates to, "Yes, please," for me. Yes, let me leave suffering behind. Yes, let us live without pain or sadness. Forever. Yes, please.
(Lyrics copyright 2002, Darrell Evans)

ABOUT THE EDITOR

Lauren Kingsland, editor, is a studio quilt artist who lives in Montgomery County, Maryland. She is the author of the classic book "The Scrapbook You Can Sleep Under". As a Visiting Artist for the Arts & Humanities program at Lombardi Comprehensive Cancer Center at Georgetown University she teaches quiltmaking as a creative outlet to patients, staff and other caregivers. Her training includes a masters degree in Applied Healing Arts from Maryland University of Integrative Health in addition to work in art, business, the humanities, classics and computer science.

"**Helping Sacred Threads 2013 become a reality has been a wonderful learning experience. Thanks everyone for being such a great team.**"

www.laurenkingsland.com

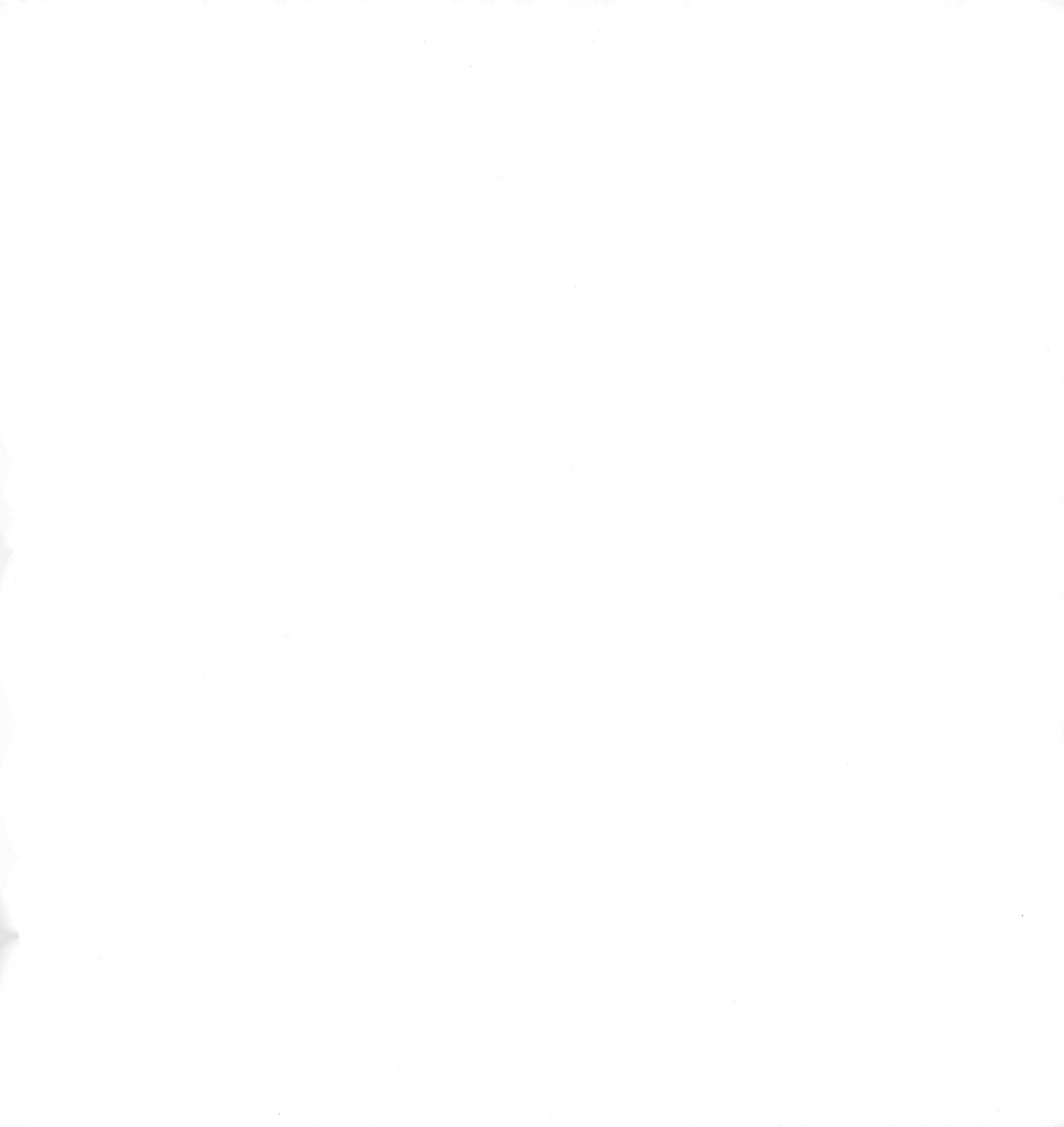

20273596R00133

Made in the USA
Charleston, SC
08 July 2013